ALCOHOL AND THE OTHER GERM POISONS

ALCOHOL

AND THE

OTHER GERM POISONS

BY

Dr. G. P. FRETS

PATHOLOGICAL ANATOMIST OF THE HOSPITAL FOR MENTAL
AND NERVOUS DISEASES AT ROTTERDAM

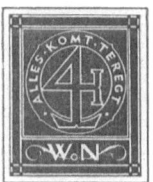

SPRINGER-SCIENCE+BUSINESS MEDIA, B.V.
1931

ISBN 978-94-017-6698-2   ISBN 978-94-017-6760-6 (eBook)
DOI 10.1007/978-94-017-6760-6

CONTENTS

TABLES:
    Tab. 1, after LAITINEN p. 11; tab. 2, Natality a. o. p. 14; tab. 3, Epilepsy p. 32; tab. 4, Imbecility p. 40; tab. 5, In-sanity p. 48; tab. 6, Alcoholism p. 52; tab. 7, after VON BUNGE, p. 56; tab. 8, after LUNDBORG p. 60; tab. 9, after FÉRÉ p. 81; tab. 10, after STOCKARD p. 87; tab. 11, after PEARL p. 90; tab. 12, after FÉRÉ p. 129.

PREFACE

A critical review from a scientific and a practical point of view is required of the significance of parental alcoholism and of the other germ poisons.

The literature on the subject is very extensive, but the problem has not been solved. The opinions on the different investigations are divided.

The publications on the other germ poisons we find spread about in the literature. In the handbooks of toxicology very little is found about them.

As to the scientific need of a study like the present, the light has repeatedly fallen on germ poisoning, especially that through alcohol by the mendelian investigations on heredity, and the question has arisen as to its value, and on the ground of those investigations the importance is sometimes doubted. Where the problem is in discussion in this way, a critical and extensive treatise of the whole literature is required.

In making this study I have adopted the critical standpoint. I have treated the subject analytically and systematically, so that in many chapters the different parts of the subject have their turn. In this way the reader can easily locate himself, and it is also shown where the weak places in our knowledge of the subject are present.

And as the literature is treated extensively, the value of the historical method appears, which somewhat enhances here the importance of earlier investigations.

Besides experimental research a large space has been devoted to medical statistical investigations. The tables will demonstrate the value of the results.

The literature has not been fully treated in this study, especially with regard to the earliest investigations nor all the parts of the problem equally extensively. In some of the publications that are dealt with here, the missing literature is mentioned.

The discussion of the other germ poisons offers the possibility of comparing the different germ poisons.

Finally, the increase of our knowledge of germ injuries by ray treatment forces us also to a comparison of its significance with that of the germ poisons.

The problem of parental alcoholism and the other germ poisons has a medical, a statistical, a biological and a sociological side. By collaboration of investigators in these different fields of work the problem will be best considered. The medical point of view will be the most important.

This is especially applicable for the practical or eugenic significance of the problem. In the various countries where an eugenic movement is developing, with the renewed appearance of alcoholism after the great war, with the increasing urgency of the problem of population, the need of eugenic reform arises and then the attention is also drawn to the alcohol problem. The question is, how far is our knowledge sufficient for practical purposes.

The author is indebted to the Dutch Physicians' Union of Total Abstainers for contributing towards the expenses incurred for the translation of the manuscript into English.

INTRODUCTION

Injuries to the germ (blastophthory) are brought about by chronic poisoning (mercury, lead, alcohol), by infection (syphilis, tuberculosis), by constitutional diseases (diseases of metabolism), by chronic underfeeding and by local diseases of the sexual glands. It may also be caused by subjection to experiments and further by ray treatment.

These injuries we know through pathologic-anatomical examinations of the sex glands of the parents, and we also conclude from examples of defective offspring that such injuries to the germ substance exist.

We consider these changes to the germ plasm to be very indefinite and they must be strictly distinguished from hereditary modifications. The question in how far acquired characters are hereditary, or may become so, will not be discussed here.

FOREL (1911) classified blastophthorical injuries to the germ as "any influence, except those of heredity, which directly and immediately disturb or destroy the structure of the cell, so that the productions of such germs, which otherwise were good in themselves, would turn out to be inferior in their further development, in consequence of a disturbance of their latent determiners (predetermined energies). If the respective determiners of the germ cells are permanently injured, this injury will without a doubt be transferred to the predisposition of the offspring and in this manner it may also happen that it will further establish itself hereditarily in their germ cells. The blastophthorical disturbances then become hereditary. Alcoholic poisoning of the germ constitutes the prototype of blastophthory."

FOREL recognises here a certain theory of heredity, which we, following our own definition, do not accept.

In connection with the possibility that mutations may arise, that is thus new hereditary variations (NILSSON-EHLE, BAUR, T. TAMMES; H. J. MÜLLER 1927, R. GOLDSCHMIDT 1929), we must bear in mind that when these might arise from the action of chemical substances (alcohol, lead) such mutations or hereditary deviations would only be seen in later generations. These changes are namely mostly recessive; if they arise as modified germ-cells then they, when fused with normal germ cells, will cause phaenotypical normal individuals to be created. Only in the following generations when two individuals which are heterozygotes for the modification mate, will the modification appear.

Of the several germ injuries named in this work only such as are caused by poisoning are dealt with.

Chemical substances, as germ poisons, may injure the new individual in three ways. The poison may affect either the male or female germ cells or the germplasm, namely before conception, or the developing germ in the various stages of development, namely after conception. Strictly speaking we discriminate between germ-cell poisoning and germ poisoning.

In the case of lead poisoning e.g., we are informed by CONSTANTIN PAUL that saturnismus of the father leads to abortion. By allowing any deleterious substance to influence the spermatozoids and the egg cells before conception, it is possible to get some idea of the difference in sensitivity of the egg-cells and spermatozoids. O. HERTWIG is of the opinion that the egg-cell is more sensitive.

By influencing the fertilised egg in different ways, DARESTE obtained many monstrosities with fowls. FÉRÉ obtained similar results by injecting all kinds of chemical substances.

In the case of man, all three effects of the germ poisons have presented themselves.

A. ALCOHOL

Of all the germ poisons, alcohol is the best known and has been investigated most. The opinion as to the signification of alcohol in this respect is very much divided. Most investigators consider alcohol as an important germ poison. There are some who doubt this significance or even reject such. Especially in the investigations of late years, we find this to be the case.

We shall endeavour to give here a critical review of the literature.

I. Data about the Use of Alcohol by Man.

Imbecility, epilepsy, insanity and malformations in children have been ascribed to parental alcoholism. Further it has been found that in cases of marriages of alcoholic parents, the number of births is greater than in families of sober habits, whilst the death rate is also higher.

The Amount of Alcohol in the Blood

In order to understand any possible effects of alcohol, such as used by man, on the germ substance, it is essential to know how alcohol stands in respect to the circulation and to the sex-glands.

The alcohol which man drinks is, for the greater part, absorbed in the stomach and the remainder in the intestines and then goes into the blood and lymph. (HANDWERK 1927).

In persons who do not drink and in mammals, alcohol is present in the blood in measureable, though very negligible quantities.

SCHWEISHEIMER found in human blood an average of 0.003 % alcohol. PRINGSHEIM found in rabbits' blood 0.002 %, in the muscles of rats 0.003 %, and in the liver 0.002 % alcohol.

KIONKA (1927) found in persons in a sober condition 0.0015—0.0127 % of alcohol in the blood, but mostly 0.0015—0.0053% and after correction an average of 0.004 %. After the consumption of a

moderate quantity of alcohol, 25 ccm abs. alcohol, he found in the
blood 0.006 %—0.016 %, an average of 0.012 % of alcohol.

HANDWERK (1927) gave larger quantities of alcohol with varying
quantities of food in the stomach. He gave for instance 2 litres of
beer (= 57 ccm abs. alcohol) and found one hour after administration an average of 0.023 % alcohol. Where he gave 4 litres (= 114
ccm abs. alcohol) he found the average quantity of alcohol in the
blood to be 0.051 % and when administering 285 ccm spirits (= 114
ccm abs. alcohol) he found somewhat less viz. 0.049 or 0.051 % alcohol in the blood. If alcoholic beverages (= 114 ccm abs. alcohol) are
taken on a full stomach, the proportion of alcohol in the blood is
distinctly lower, viz. 0.024 %.

A small part 5 % of the alcohol which is absorbed by the stomach
and intestines and taken up by the blood, is secreted by the kidneys.
If the quantity of urine is increased (after taking coffee etc.) the percentage of alcohol passed by the kidneys is higher; the degree of alcohol in the blood is in any case lower. (PFEIFER 1927).

French investigators have found higher values with animals.

NICLOUX (1900) is of the opinion that there may be traces of alcohol
in normal blood but these minute quantities are of no importance with
regard to the quantity which is found after alcohol has been used.

NICLOUX (1899) in his experiments on pregnant guinea pigs gave
10 % alcohol through the stomach tube. He gave 5 ccm pure alcohol
per 1 kilo animal weight and found in the blood 0.36 % alcohol and
in the blood of the foetus 0.31. When he gives 1 ccm he finds resp.
0.13 % and 0.08 %. He had similar results with dogs and sheep.

In the case of pregnant women, he found that if he gave 60 ccm of
rum with 45 % alcohol, which is equivalent to $\frac{1}{2}$ ccm pure alcohol per
1 kilo weight of body, there was an average of 0.03 % alcohol in the
blood taken from the umbilical cord.

GRÉHANT (1900) found when administering 1 ccm pure alcohol per
kilo animal weight into the stomach of a dog, 0.13 % pure alcohol in
the blood. When administering 6 ccm per kilo body weight the animal
became unconscious and insensible and then he found 0.7 % pure alcohol. After 23 hours there was no trace of alcohol in the blood. The
largest dosage which GRÉHANT gave is 10 ccm per kilo body weight
and then the maximum proportion of alcohol is 1.08 %, $2\frac{3}{4}$ hours
after the beginning of the test. When GRÉHANT (1899) gave a dog a

still larger dose of alcohol (22.2 ccm abs. alc. pro kilo bodyweight) the animal dies. GRÉHANT found consecutively 1.1 %, 1.35 % and 1.42% abs. alcohol in the blood. In the organs of man 0.3—0.4 % alcohol has been found (cit. TRIBOULET 1922).

KOBERT (1906 II, page 936) states that in cases of animals highly narcotized by alcohol, 0.72 % alcohol is found in the blood and 0.12 % when there is only lethargy. See also ROGER (1922, p. 25).

According to an article by VIEILLEDENT (1926) 4—6 % of alcohol in the blood would cause death by alcoholic poisoning, 2—4 % would bring about drunkenness. These are improbably high figures. In cases of drunkenness the lowest observation is 4 per thousand. The individual factor is of importance. In acute cases of alcoholic poisoning in man an alcohol concentration of 0.33 % is found in the blood according to PAUL and BONNE (cit. HOPPE).

Alcohol in the Cerebro-Spinal Fluid

SCHOTMÜLLER and SCHUMM (1912) examined with the aid of the LIEBEN iodoform test, the liquor cerebrospinalis for alcohol in a number of alcoholics after their admittance into the hospital. The result with two patients was negative, but with several it was distinctly positive. The utility of the iodoform test at these examinations was criticised by VORKÄSTNER and NEUE (1913). SCHOTMÜLLER and SCHUMM (1913) replying to this said that with the test with persons who had not used alcohol shortly before, the result was negative. In the meantime the authors have been successful in quantitatively defining alcohol in the liquor cerebrospinalis. In one instance SCHOTMÜLLER found 0.8 % of alcohol in the distillate. NICLOUX when experimenting with guinea pigs and dogs found 0.4 % alcohol in the cerebrospinal fluid and 0.4 % in the blood. The animals received 5 ccm pure alcohol per kilo body weight.

Alcohol in the Mother's Milk

Older investigators, BAER, BESSEY and DEMME mention the transmission of alcohol in the milk and see in this the possibility of an influence on the suckling through the use of alcohol by the mother. The existence of idiocy and imbecility is explained in this way by BESSEY. DEMME informs us that a child suckled by an alco-

holic mother — she drank daily 200/250 grammes of spirits — suffered from severe convulsions which subsided as soon as the child was
fed with other milk.

KLINGEMANN (1891) undertook experiments with four goats. He
found if they were given a little alcohol (up to 50 ccm) no alcohol
could be traced in the milk. If a larger dosage (100/200 ccm) was
given, then small quantities passed over into the milk but not more
than 0.5 % of the alcohol given.

ROSEMANN (1900) came to the same result in his experiments with
cows and likewise KOLDEWYN (1910) who just like KLINGEMANN
gave alcohol to a goat in the food and through the stomach tube. Only when the body was suddenly supplied with a large quantity of
alcohol was there a small quantity found in the milk. One day after
use alcohol was no longer found in the milk. KOLDEWYN does not
mention NICLOUX's experiments (see below).

The former results are contradictory to the experience in the
clinics. (DEMME 1890, page 82). E. TOULOUSE (1891, 1896, page 50)
and MUSKENS (1924 page 311) for instance remind us of how small
quantities of alcohol consumed by the nurse cause the baby to react
with convulsions.

NICLOUX (1899) gave a wetnurse 60 ccm rum, thus $\frac{1}{2}$ ccm pure
alcohol per kilo bodyweight and found 0.07 % alcohol in the milk;
in a second experiment he found 0.08% alcohol. NICLOUX (1900)
when giving dogs 3 ccm pure alcohol per kilo animal weight, found in
the mother's milk 0.25 % alcohol. Making another experiment by
giving 4 ccm pure alcohol he then found 0.37 % in the blood and
0.27 % in the milk. NICLOUX finds in his method no alcohol in the
milk of the suckling woman, who does not take alcohol. When
experimenting with a sheep he found 0.2 % alcohol in the milk.

NICLOUX is of the opinion that convulsions in sucklings are to be
ascribed to the use of alcohol on the part of the wetnurse.

Alcohol in the Blood of the Placenta; in the Amnion Fluid;
in the Sperm. Congenital Alcoholism

NICLOUX (1900) made many investigations about the proportion of
alcohol in the blood and tissues (page 4).

He also investigated the proportion of alcohol in the placenta and in the amnion liquid and on the basis of the positive findings of this investigation he differentiates congenital alcoholism.

He found (1899) in the blood of the placenta of women 0.03 % alcohol. In the amnion water of the foetus he found 0.46 % alcohol (there was 0.5 % in the mother's blood); in another experiment these figures were 0.22 and 0.3 % respectively.

In the testicles of the guinea pig or the dog he found 0.2 % (in the blood 0.3 %); in a further experiment these figures were 0.4 and 0.48 % respectively. Similar figures were also found for the ovaries.

NICLOUX found in the sperm of man — the experimental person having imbibed 1.5 ccm abs. alcohol per 1 kilo body weight — 0.11 % alcohol. (In the blood the percentage was calculated at 0.15 %).

The cells of the body therefore, the germ cells as well, are all in contact with the alcohol which the person consumes as a beverage. The quantity is indicative of the quantity of alcohol used.

Toxic and Lethal Dose.

The venom of alcoholic beverages concerns the aethylalcohol itself and the admixtures (VON JAKSCH 1910, BUMKE 1914).

The lethal dosage for non-drinkers according to TAILOR is 60—180 grammes, according to KUNKEL 100—200 grammes (cited by KOBERT 1906; see also page 4).

a. Pathological-anatomical Alterations of the Germ-glands

Pathological-anatomical changes of the sexual glands are especially known from the investigations of SIMMONDS (1898, 1910), of BERTHOLET (1909, 11) of WEICHSELBAUM and KYRLE (1912) and of KYRLE and SCHOPPER (1914; early literature).

BERTHOLET examined the testicles at 210 post mortem examinations among which were 100 bodies of chronic alcoholics. WEICHSELBAUM and KYRLE reported more than 57 cases, later then a further 18 cases. The latter were specially investigated because the liver showed no signs of modifications to which the changes in the testicles might be attributed. Atrophy of the testicles, fatty degeneration of the gland cells and an increase of the connective tissues was noticed.

There are different grades of alterations. Finally no more sperm cells were traced. SIMMONDS also finds azoospermia.

WEICHSELBAUM and KYRLE are of the opinion that besides degenerative changes, there are also signs of regeneration. BERTHOLET examined two cases where total abstinence of more than 25 years had succeeded alcoholism. In this instance regeneration and normal sperm cells were found.

BERTHOLET examined some females and found in the ovaries changes corresponding to those of the males in the testicles. (LANCERAUX likewise had the same experience, cit. TRIBOULET).

BERTHOLET thinks that in cases where fatty degeneration of the gland cells is met with, but where moreover, numerous spermatozoids are present, children with reduced resistance, with feeblemindedness and malformations are born.

WEICHSELBAUM points out that especially in cases of chronic alcoholism where cirrhosis of the liver is found, changes in the testicles are met with. BERTHOLET, found changes stronger where tuberculosis was present at the same time. It is possible with chronic alcoholism that there is some connection between constitutional and germ cell degeneration.

KYRLE and SCHOPPER (1914) examined the liver and testicles of rabbits which they had given alcohol. Large quantities were given which were equal to a daily consumption of $\frac{1}{4}$ litre 50 % gin of a person of 80 kilos weight. They report on 31 rabbits. They found in the testicles an irregular atrophy with a slight local increase of the interstitial tissue.

WELLER (1930) found similar changes with cases of acute alcoholism.

BONIN and GARNIER (1900) gave diluted alcohol as daily food to white rats and found in two instances after 8 and 11 months respectively important anatomical changes in the testicles. The seminiferous tubes were narrower and the epithelium in some places had almost disappeared. There was cell degeneration but there were no vascular changes. Few spermatozoids were found. There were also some nucleus divisions with the spermatoblasts and signs of amitosis, attempts of yet unripe spermatides to transform themselves into spermatozoids. The spermatozoids were the most sensitive of the different forms of development. Before they degenerated some were still able to fertilise. This would explain the deviations in the offspring of alcoholics (cf. BERTHOLET page 8). Degeneration and regeneration which is found in the testicles of alcoholics is also found in the testicles of animals after ray treatment (HERXHEIMER 1926).

ARLITT and WELLS (1917) examined the sexual glands of rats where alcohol had been added to the food. During life unhealthy indications were noticed and of the organs examined only the testicles showed marked anatomical changes. There was a decrease in the size and also the seminiferous tubes were smaller and the number of spermatozoids had decreased; there was no interstitial inflammation. The result of the examination of the ovaries is uncertain.

C. GRAVE found in albino rats of HANSON and HANDY treated wiht inhalation of alcoholic fumes (17 months, 6 of each 7 days, $\frac{1}{2}$—4 hours) that testes and ovaries show a marked departure from the normal appearance. STOCKARD did not find any changes. See also KOSTITSCH p. 97, and STIEVE, p. 125.

In judging the changes named herein there is some room for difference of opinion; there are those who are not convinced. In general one need only pursue the manuals on pathological anatomy (e.g. HERXHEIMER 1919, page 811, II 1164, 1103; KAUFFMANN 1922) in which it is inferred that in cases of chronic alcoholism these changes of the sexual glands occur.

VON JAKSCH (1910 page 291) in his judgment says that one can easily determine the anatomical diagnosis of chronic alcoholism from the joint anatomical changes of the different organs which is found in every occurrent case. Here it must further be taken into consideration that alcohol belongs to the group of poisons which in acute cases causing death does not show marked changes of the internal organs (KOBERT 1906).

b. Clinical and Statistical Data

Many data are found in the alcohol literature and also in medical works.

BUMKE, the Director of the Psychiatric Clinics at Munich, writes for example in 1924 in his manual on mental diseases: "Alcohol reduces the number of viable children; miscarriages and stillbirths are frequent in alcoholic families and a large number of the children born alive die in the first year from convulsions, general impairment or in consequence of very slight resistance against infectious diseases." At an examination of the clinics at Munich BUMKE informs us that it was found that with a group of serious alcoholics, the total number of children alive did not reach the total number of parents as long as they were still alive.

Older workers who ascertained the injurious effects of alcohol on human offspringg are MARTIN (1897), DÉJÉRINE (1886), DEMME (1890), ANTON (1901), LAITINEN (1909) and many others. We shall now discuss consecutively the various injuries to children of alcoholic parents named in the literature.

1. Natality and Infantile Mortality; Body Weight

ARRIVÉE (1899) made in France a demographic study of about 1600 confinements and divided them into 3 groups. The first comprised 433 cases of alcoholic parents, the second 368 cases of tuberculous parents and the third group 847 other cases. ARRIVÉE found abortus in 50 cases of the alcohol group i.e. 11.5 %, in the tuberculous group 35 cases i.e. 9.8 % and in the undefined group 56 cases i.e. 6.6 %. There were 13 premature births in 363 confinements of alcoholics i.e. 3.6 % and in the undefined group the percentage is 0.64 %. ARRIVÉE found in the group with alcoholic heredity 20 cases of stillborn at 383 confinements i.e. 5.2 % of the cases, 3.6 % of the group tuberculous heredity and in the undefined group 2.8 %.

The infantile mortality in the first group (alcoholic heredity) is 112 deaths in the first year out of 363 births and 53 deaths between the first and fifth year, together 167 deaths from 0 to 5 years of age i.e. 46 %. The number of deaths in the case of 791 children in the first five years and from healthy parents aggregated 25.4 %.

The infant mortality mentioned in the material of MARTIN's (see page 19) and that of LANCERAUX (page 19) is great.

LEGRAIN (1895) found among 814 children of drinkers 174 cases of premature birth, stillborn, infantile mortality together i.e. 21 %, a much lower percentage than ARRIVÉE.

SULLIVAN (1900) gives the following information about infantile mortality with alcoholics. Of 120 female inebriates were born 600 children, of whom 335 (55.8 per cent) died under two years, or were dead born. In over 60% of the children dying in infancy the assigned cause of death was convulsions. SULLIVAN gives the following standard of comparison. Drunken mothers (21 cases) had 125 children, of which 69 (55.2%) died under 2 years. Sober mothers (28 cases) had 138 children of which 33 (23.9%) died under 2 years.

SULLIVAN (1900) finds a progressive death rate in the alcoholic family classing the children in the order of their birth.

For statistical study of the question of the significance of parental alcoholism one must rely on simple and known material. The best thing is that investigators collect their own material.

The work of Prof. LAITINEN (1909) of Helsingfors has the advantage that for many years as a physician with a large practice, he made observations himself, alcoholic families were compared with sober families. In his investigations three groups of observations are named which on account of the agreement of the results which may be deduced therefrom increase their significance.

In the first place LAITINEN mentions the results of the study of data which were obtained by investigations in a small town. (tab. 1)

	50 sober families	50 alcoholic families
Housing; Average number of rooms . .	2.83	2.31
Average age mother	39.52 years	39 years
„ „ father	47.16 „	40.27 „
„ number of children per family	4.28	4.72
Number of children deceased in youth .	18.48 %	24.82 %
Still alive	81.52 %	75 %
Miscarriages	0.94 %	6.21 %
Weak at birth	1.3 %	8.27 %
Convulsions first years	. . . .	3.23 %

One would perhaps like to know here as well as in the following groups whether one or both parents were total abstainers, also whether roughly in both groups there are as many families with one or two children (page 16); yet the fact that LAITINEN knows his material thoroughly and investigated a part himself, makes the reliability of the results very great.

The second group is the result of sending out a circular. 1285 parental alcoholics (623 moderate, 662 heavy) and 840 sober parents sent in details asked for about the weight of sucklings which were weighed every week for 8 months, and also about aliments and teething. The children about which details were given were as a rule the third or fourth child and the data covers 840 children of non-drinking parents, 623 children of moderate drinkers and 622 of heavier drinkers. Moderate drinkers are those who do not consume more alcohol per day than that contained in a glass of beer (4% alcohol).

The conditions of life, the age and the housing conditions were roughly about the same in the 3 groups. The weight of the children of sober parents was always greatest. The average number of teeth of eight months old children of sober parents was greatest, the number of children of such parents, which were without teeth was the smallest, the average age when the first tooth was cut was the lowest for children of sober parents.

The results in the case of children of moderate drinking parents always fluctuates between those of non-alcoholic parents and harder drinking parents.

In the third place LAITINEN has at his disposal his own observations in 3611 families with 17094 children. The mean weight of body at birth of the whole material is greatest in children (boys as well as girls) of sober parents. From LAITINEN's own material the number of children per family is by far the greatest of parents who are hard drinkers, in moderate drinking parents the average number of children is smaller and in parents of temperate habits the average is also smaller. The death rates of children in the same order in LAITINEN's material are 32 %, 23 % and 13.5 %, the number of miscarriages 7 %, 5 % and 1 %.

LAITINEN's material therefore presents a greater infantile death rate and a greater average number of children per family in alcoholic families. The weight of the child at birth and the development in the first year is more favourable in children of non-drinkers than in those of intemperate parents.

PEARSON and ELDERTON (1910) show divergent results in their well known statistical investigations. They do not find any difference in the weight of those children attending schools in the poorest part of Edinburgh, in the height of children of parents where the father drinks and only a noticeable difference if the mother drinks. They examined 315 sons and 270 daughters of parents who drank and 207 daughters of parents who did not drink.

There is a higher death rate among offspring of alcoholic than among offspring of non-alcoholic parents; the families in the former case are larger. This applies to the material for Edinburgh as well as for Manchester. On these points, the mean weight of the children and the death rate, PEARSON's results do not differ from LAITINEN's. PEARSON also refers to this himself (2nd. study page 19). He writes "We have noticed a different ratio in weight of an equally slight character and a substantial difference in mortality."

The result of the investigations as to the health of the children in connection with the use of alcohol on the part of parents gives rise to some doubt as to the suitability of the material for the problem investigated. For children attending schools for backward children in Manchester the authors find normal health in sons in a slightly larger number in the case where the father or the mother drinks than if they do not drink; in the case of daughters the results for both groups differ. The differences are so slight as to be of no importance. As this particular school is attended only by children of families in which at least one child is mentally deficient, the question arises as to the state of the health of the parents who do not drink. Nothing is mentioned of this.

The number of children suffering from tuberculosis and epilepsy in the material for Manchester is greater in the case of sober parents than of alcoholic parents.

As to intellectual development here PEARSON also finds the percentage of mentally normal children smaller with moderate drinking parents than with immoderate. This result is clearer for Manchester than for Edinburgh; he writes: "Here again we must repeat that we do not suppose temperance to be a cause of mental defect any more than we suppose it should be a cause of phtisis or epilepsy. The slight association, if it be significant, is probably a secondary effect of an hereditary influence, the mentally defective children coming from a feebler stock, which has not the desire or possibly the capacity for alcohol of a stock of a more vigorous physique." Indeed one would like to know the parents i.e. something of the genotype of the children.

It is possible that in the material mental defectiveness, tuberculosis,

TABLE 2. PARENTAL ALCOHOLISM AND NATALITY, ABORTION, MORTALITY, MORBIDITY [1]

	Authors	Drinkers			Indifferent			Teetotallers		
		N. of cases	N. of Deviations	%	N. of cases	N. of Deviations	%	N. of cases	N. of Deviations	%
Natality	LAITINEN	59	4.72 [2]					50	4.28 [2]	
(size of family)	SICHEL	120	4.71 [2]							
"	SULLIVAN	120	5 [2]					28	4.93 [2]	
Body weight at birth	LUNDBORG		5.6 [2]			4.9 [2]				
" " "	LAITINEN	with teetotallers the greatest								
" " "	PEARSON and ELDERTON	with drinking parents smaller than with sober ones.								
Abortion	ARRIVÉE	433	50	11.5	847	56	6.6			
"	LAITINEN	often						less often.		
"	MINOR	1064 [3]	1513							
"	POLISCH	170	23	13.5						
Premature birth	ARRIVÉE	363	13	3.6			0.64			
Stillborn	BOSS (1929)	383	20	5.2			2.8			
"	BOSS (1929)	1246		6						
mortality 0—1 yr.	ARRIVÉE	363	112	30						
1—5 "	"		53							
0—5 "	"	363	167	46	791		25.4	138	33	23.9
0—2 "	SULLIVAN	600	335	55.8						
0—2 "	BOSS	1246		7						
Died young	MARTIN 1879	244	132	54	83 [4]	37	45			
Young mortality	LANCERAUX 1879	410	169	41						
"	LAITINEN			24.8			23.2			18.5
"	BUMKE 1924	many		32						13.5
"	PEARSON and ELDERTON	with drinking parents greater than with sober ones.								

„	Jörger (Zero)	300	74	24
„	Demme			24
„	Rosenberg	great		
„	Lundborg	great		
„ 0—2 yr.	Preisig and Amadian . .	613		23
„ 0—1 yr.	Plaut 1909	183		32.7
„ 0—1 yr.	Polisch 1927 [5] . . .	170	24	14
„	Panse 1929	720		18
Premature birth stillborn and young mortality	Legrain 1895	814	174	21
Still born and died young	Stuchlik 1915	50	13	26
morbidity	Martin 1879	inferior nervous system page 19.		
„	Allers 1911	great baby mortality coincides with great infant mortality and less fitness for military service (Cf. p. 16).		
„	Sichel 1910	247	42	17 [6]
„	Stuchlik 1915	50	22	44 [7]
„	Plaut 1909			59

[1]) With the investigation by the League of Nations after the causes of the baby mortality (1930) 4 groups are distinguished: 1 low mortality 3.6—4.7 %; still births 2.9—3.7 %; 2 mediocre mortality 5.2—6.4 %; still births 2.4—4.0 %; 3. high morality 7.6—9.8 %; still births 1.6—6.4 %; and 4. very high mortality 10.6—19.8 %; still births 2.6—3.9 %.

[2]) Size of family.   [3]) Families.   [4]) parental alcoholism not certain or failing.

[5]) Marriages of male sufferers from delirium tremens.

[6]) great number of defective and unhealthy children and moreover great infantile mortality. (Sichel).

[7]) includes stillbirths, died young, and the sick.

and epilepsy are present from other causes than from alcohol, which make the effects of alcohol invisible.

PEARSON (1911) criticized LAITINEN's work. The methods for statistics were not always properly applied. We must acknowledge, that this should be taken into account. The very first consideration however is that the material is serviceable for the purpose. One must know the material and it must be simply compiled. In this respect the investigations of LAITINEN's are of greater value than PEARSON's. (See also page 31—36).

In contradiction to the opinion of PEARSON and of PEARL (page 87) that alcoholism may have a selective effect by reason of the increased death rate of children, ALLERS (1911, page 656) states that in general always in our civilised territories, territories with a high death rate of babies coincide with those of a large infantile mortality and those of a smaller number of persons fit for military service.

According to D. HERON's investigations on the feeble-minded inebriate, these alcoholic women two thirds of whom are mentally defective had not smaller but larger families than sound stocks, 865 female inebriates had in all 2589 children.

A higher death rate among children is always found where the mother is alcoholic. SULLIVAN ascertained in alcoholic mothers a mortality among the offspring up to the end of the second year of 55.8 %. The children mostly died of convulsions (cit. V. WLASSAK 1929).

SICHEL (1910) names 100 married patients emanating from alcoholic families, 22 marriages were childless, nothing was known of 10 marriages, and of the remaining number with a total of 565 children, 200 children died, 205 were healthy, 118 are alive but the state of their health is unknown, and 142 are ailing and defective i.e. 25 % (see also page 37). The mean size of family is 4.71 children in 120 marriages; the death rate is 35.4 %. Of the 247 children of which the condition of health was unknown, 205 were healthy and 42 ill and defective i.e. 17 % ailing. MINOR (1911) found in 1064 families where either the men or women were treated for alcoholism (see also page 50) 1513 miscarriages. STUCHLICK (1915) found in the material of the Psychiatric Clinics at Zurich that of 50 children of married alcoholics (page 69) only 28 (56 %) were healthy, 13 (26 %) stillborn or died at an early age. KRAEPELIN (1909) informs us of the result of investiga-

tions by PLAUT. 32.7 % of 183 children of alcoholics died in their
first year and 59 % of the survivors were not physically sound.
Further nearly half of the remainder showed signs of bodily disorder
and disturbed development.

In the Zero family (cf. page 61) the natality and mortality were
both high. Of the 300 Zeros 74 died in infancy i.e. 24 %, the same
percentage as DEMME found (tab. 2).

ROSENBERG also reports a high death rate among children. Increased fertility and high death rate among children is reported by
LUNDBORG (see also page 62). ELIASSOW (1915) finds in families of
children attending a school for defectives an infant death rate of 30.9%
(see page 38). PREISIG and AMADIAN found among 613 children of
100 cured alcoholics an infant mortality of 23 % (under two years),
which does not differ from the general death tables in Switzerland.
The physical and psychological condition of children is not unfavourable (page 69).

POLISCH (1927c) found among 170 cases of gravidity in 58 marriages
with male delirants, 23 cases of abortion, 1 stillborn and 23 deaths in
the first year (15 %). The 8 cases where the marriages were childless
are not included in this material. The infant death rate according to
the annual returns does not differ from that of Berlin in the same
year (20—11 %). In 7 out of 23 deaths of babies convulsions were the
cause. POLISCH refers to the little value of this report of the parents
(see also V. WLASSAK, 1929 page 137).

Boss (1929) in his material of alcoholics finds with female drinkers
twice as many abortions and still-birth and three times as great a
baby mortality as with non-drinkers.

The wives of 489 drinkers have 1246 births, among which are 6 %
stillborns and 7 % deaths in the first two years. These figures are low
and not higher than in the general population.

From table 2 (p. 14, 15) we see: —

The mean number of children per family of drinking parents is larger than with sober parents.

The mean body weight at birth of children of alcoholic parents is
smaller than with children of sober parents.

The number of abortions, premature births and still births is larger
with drinking than with sober parents. This appears, for instance,
when comparing the figures by ARRIVÉE. The value of his figures

can be judged well, because the author has examined both alcoholics and non-alcoholics (cf also SULLIVAN).

The mortality among children of drinking parents is very high. The figures of different authors differ here very much. Illnesses are more frequent with children of drinking parents than with children of non-drinking parents. The physical and mental condition of the latter is not so good. The figures here are also divergent. Moreover, some authors obtained other results (ELDERTON and PEARSON). On degeneration see page 64.

2. Epilepsy

In the textbooks of mental and nervous diseases and in monographs on epilepsy the great significance of alcoholism of the parents in respect to epilepsy in the children is always referred to. I refer to ECHEVERRIA (1881), DÉJÉRINE (1886), FÉRÉ (1890), E. TOULOUSE (1896), O. BINSWANGER (1899), KRAEPELIN (1913), REDLICH (1924), MUSKENS (1924), JELGERSMA (1926), BUMKE (1924), NOTKIN (1928), LANGE (1927) and many others. Extensive literature is referred to by STÜBER (1921).

It must be remembered when we see that alcoholic parents have inferior children, that alcohol may be the cause of this in three ways. In the first place as a manifestation of heredity, secondly as a manifestation of germ poisoning and thirdly by insufficient care given to children in a family where the father, and still more so where the mother is addicted to drink.

Very much importance is always attached to the significance of heredity. Especially in the sense that we are of the opinion that persons predisposed to be defective become alcoholics „ne devient pas alcoholiste qui ne veut" (LASÈGUE), and that therefore many defectives are found among children of alcoholics.

Besides this alcohol has also a poisonous effect on the germ. O. BINSWANGER (1899) understands by hereditary transmission of epilepsy, not only or in the first place the psychopatic constitution of the parents, but lays stress on all illnesses which seriously harm the state of nutrition of the parents. Of these the most investigated are alcoholism, syphilis, tuberculosis and gout. These illnesses have therefore an injurious effect as germ poison. KRAEPELIN (1913) also

considers that epilepsy, at least to the same extent, is the expression
of a germ injury as of hereditary transmission. JELGERSMA (1926)
(III 476) is of the same opinion.

Of the many investigations made concerning the aetiology of epilepsy in which attention is also drawn to alcohol, the following may
be mentioned.

MOREAU (1854) found in relatives of 364 epileptics, 250 cases of bad
health including 30 cases of epilepsy, 24 cases of alcoholism, 25 cases
of convulsions, 26 cases of insanity, 35 cases of tuberculosis. MOREAU
arrives at a percentage of 19.35 % alcoholic parents with 124 epileptics, from his own material.

A. VOISIN (1883) found out of 95 ordinary epileptics 12.6 % with
ancestors who died from alcoholic excess.

H. MARTIN (1879) finds that alcoholism of the parents is very frequently a cause of convulsions in the first year and of epilepsy in
their descendants. MARTIN investigated the cases of epileptic patients
in the Salpetriere in 1874; there where 130/150. MARTIN had very
good family data of 83 epileptic patients. Of 60 of these patients, the
use of alcohol by the parents is positive, but with the remaining 23 it
was doubtful. It is of importance that MARTIN gave a brief description of the illness in 12 of his cases. The 60 epileptic patients had 244
brothers and sisters, 48 of whom had convulsions in the first year
(20 %), 132 died young (54 %); of the 112 survivors some had a
weak nervous system. Most of them were still very young when the
observations were made; this explains that no alcoholics are mentioned among them. The 23 epileptic patients, where parental alcoholism
was not certain or was lacking, had 83 brothers and sisters, 10 of
which had convulsions (12 %) and 37 died young (45 %). The percentages in the second group are therefore somewhat lower.

Among the parents and grandparents of the total number of 83
epileptic patients, the following illnesses and causes of death were
named: — 60 cases of alcoholism as stated before, 15 cases of apo-
plexy, 5 cases of heart disease, 4 cases of suicide, 5 cases of hysterics
and 4 cases of insanity and dementia. MARTIN remarks here that the
number of cases of insanity and of epilepsy is small

MARTIN is finally of the opinion that of the surviving children of
inebriate parents, no less than one third become epileptic.

LANCERAUX (1879) reports of 83 families observed by him, in

which one or more members suffered from d iseases of alcoholic origin. There were 410 children. Of this number 1 08 (more than one fourth) had convulsions and in 1874, 169 were de ad (41 %) and 241 living, but 83 (more than a third of the survivors) were epileptic. (see tables 2 and 3).

Déjérine (1889) has defined alcoholism in the ascending line of 350 epileptic patients (108 males and 242 females) of the service of Bourneville's at Bicêtre and at la Salpétrière. He found in 51.6 % of the cases alcoholism, 2.8 % in the mother, and 37.7 % in the father, 12 % in the grandfather, 2.4 % in the grandmother and 0.4 % in other relatives. Déjérine observes that it is certainly very difficult to detemine alcoholism only on the basis of information obtained at later dates (page 114, page 98). Fêré (1890) has also investigated the heredity of epileptic patients of the Salpétrière and Bicêtre. He found in 308 male epileptics alcoholism in 62 cases in the male line and 56 times in the female line i.e. 38.3 % of the cases. Of 286 epileptic females Féré found alcoholism 72 times in the male line and 58 times in the female line i.e. 45.4 % of the cases. Bournéville (1901) informs us of the occurrence of parental alcoholism in patients admitted by him in the years 1879—1900, suffering from epilepsy, hysterics and idiocy. Of the total number of 2554 patients received, 2072 males and 482 females, he found in 785 boys and 148 girls paternal alcoholism; in 67 boys and 13 girls maternal alcoholism and in 30 boys and 10 girls alcoholism of both parents. Of 17.8 % of the patients no family data were available and in 41.1 % of the patients there was no parental alcoholism. E. Toulouse (1896) reports the views of French clinicians and observes that the children of alcoholics are epileptics, idiots and imbeciles, sufferers from different psychoses and from hysterics. Triboulet and Mignot (1922), the authors of the chapter on alcoholism in the New Medical Manual of Roger, Widal and Teissier have taken up a similar standpoint.

Among the writers on aetiology of epilepsy Echeverria (1880) is always referred to. Also concerning the significance of parental alcoholism in respect to that aetiology. He made clinical statistical investigations (1881). Echeverria was physician-inchief to the Hospital for Epileptics and Paralytics and to the City Asylum for the insane, New York. He reports on 572 individuals affected with alcoholic epilepsy. The first division of his material contains 257 cases, 140 males and 117 females with alcoholism and epilepsy in clear sequential relationship. Of 139 patients, 75 males and 64 females, ECHEVERRIA was able to obtain particulars of the habits and nervous affections of the parents. These 139 cases comprise 92 in which intemperance either alone or associated with epilepsy existed among the parents. In the remaining 42 cases, the tendency to alcoholic excess with resultant epilepsy was inherited from insane or epileptic parents who sprung, at least some of them (seven fathers and nine mothers) from hard drinking parents.

This material of ECHEVERRIA is complicated owing to the patients suffering from epilepsy and alcoholism at the same time. In the ascending line of these patients more alcoholism will be found than in the ascending line of patients suffering from epilepsy alone. ECHEVERRIA referring to his material points out that in the ascending line of alcoholics, alcoholism occurs with insanity, epilepsy and nervous diseases and that these diseases may be found alternately in the different generations (page 18 and page 31—36). When considering the total of 572 alcoholic epileptics, ECHEVERRIA found parental intemperance alone in 18.2% of the males and in 16.2% of the females; parental intemperance attended with epilepsy or insanity existed in 16 % of the males and in 19.2 % of the females. ECHEVERRIA concludes that the extent of epilepsy in the progeny of intemperate individuals reaches 20.25 % and he finds a ratio of 17.2 intemperate parents among ordinary epileptics. There is roughly the same percentage of alcoholics in the ascending line of epileptics and of epilepsy in the descending line of alcoholics (page 35). For this reason ECHEVERRIA says that it is only fair to regard 18 % as very near the real proportion of cases of epilepsy arising from intemperance in the parents not accompanied with mental or nervous diseases.

DEMME (1890) found in 71 cases of epilepsy in the children's hospital at Berne, 21 cases of alcoholism of parents i.e. 30 %. In another group of 27 cases he found 8 cases of alcoholism of parents i.e. also 30%. In the first series there were moreover 9 epileptic fathers and 3 mothers. DEMME found in 17 cases alcoholism still further in the ascending line.

Among 814 children of drinkers LEGRAIN (1895) found 173 cases of convulsions (22.7 %) in the first year and 131 times (17.2 %) epilepsy and hysterics. Of the children of female drunkards 219 lived

beyond infancy and of these nine, or 4.1%, became epileptic according to SULLIVAN (1900).

20.5 % of the psychotic patients of the material of KOLLER
(1895, see also page 43) with alcoholic heredity are especially patients with alcoholic psychoses, epilepsy and congenital mental
deficiencies (imbeciles and idiots). In case of alcoholic epileptics
BRATZ (1899) found with 44 out of 50 patients roughly 88 % with hereditary transmission. In 16 of these patients the hereditary factor
was alcoholism of father (32 %); 4 of these had epileptic brothers and
sisters. SICHEL (1910) found among 308 patients admitted into the
Asylum at Frankfort on Main in 1907 and 1908 where excessive use
of alcohol on the part of the parents was reported, 15.2 % suffering
from epilepsy. Of the 276 admissions (from the same material as
above) for epilepsy, hysterics and imbecility he found 166 cases i.e.
16 % due to parental alcoholism.

BRATZ (1908) confirms the results of SICHEL, who found in his
material for Frankfort few Jews and that with Jewish epileptics
there was little alcoholism in the ascending line. BRATZ found in Berlin among 1262 epileptics observed by him, 28 Jews i.e. $2\frac{1}{2}$ %. In
Berlin there is a Jewish population of 10 %. With these 28 epileptic
Jews BRATZ did not find any instances of alcoholism of the parents,
whilst of 1234 non-Jewish patients, 254 showed alcoholic heredity,
mostly of the father. He finds in his material 589 times no hereditary
transmission, 391 times neuropathy and 254 times alcoholism. He
also found with hysterics alcoholism in the ascending line. In Japan
MYAKE (cit. BRATZ) found with dementia praecox 4 % potators in the
ascendency (page 46).

GRIFFITH (1911) found in 154 cases, 8 of parental alcoholism thus
only 5.2 % of the cases. O. BINSWANGER (1899) has at his disposal
information of 121 cases concerning heredity out of 150 cases of
epilepsy. In 26 cases he found alcoholism in the ascending line i.e.
22 % (17 in case of the father, 2 of the mother, 4 of the grandfather
and 3 of other members of the family).

Alcoholism of the parents as the only hereditary cause was found
by BINSWANGER in 8 cases (6.5 %). These would be certain cases
of germ injury. GALLE a pupil of BINSWANGER found in such material not favourable for family investigations, only 12 cases of drunkenness of the father or of the mother in 607 male epileptics. BINS-

WANGER observes that there is very little alcoholism in Thuringia.

KRAEPELIN (1913) found in 303 cases of epilepsy of males, 18.2 % caused by parental intemperance, in 104 cases of females, 19.2 % and 267 cases of patients under 20 years, 21 %.

VOLLAND found in the material of 24 families with epileptic brothers and sisters 4 with hereditary antecedants of mental disease, epilepsy and alcoholism simultaneously and moreover three cases of alcoholism of the father only. MUNSON (1911 page 343) found in 78 cases of traumatic epilepsy 39 times alcoholism in the direct ascending line and further 23 cases in other collateral relatives.

E. MÜLLER (1910, 1911) can show in the material of the 503 cases in the Hospital for Epileptics at Zurich during 1896/1907, 171 cases of alcoholism thus 34 % (epilepsy 10 %, psychoses and neuroses 29.2 %). GRENIER (cit. E. MÜLLER) examined the children of 188 alcoholics; in 43 of these cases there was also mental derangement with the alcoholism; 145 were alcoholics alone. Of 195 children there were 98 i. e. 52 % alcoholics, 69 i.e. 36.7 % had delirium tremens and 143 i.e. 73 % were suffering from convulsions of which 46, i.e. 24 % from epilepsy.

NEUMANN (cit. E. MÜLLER) calculated from several statistics that 16.4 of the children of drinkers suffered from epilepsy and that in 23.7 % of the cases of epilepsy, parental lacoholism in the ascending line was found.

ROSENBERG (1913) finds no connection in the 8 cases in his material between epilepsy and parental alcoholism (see page 61). STÜBER (1921) gives a compilation from the literature (his tables page 379) on hereditary alcoholism of epileptics which shows a mean figure of 33 %.

DAVENPORT and WEEKS (1911) collected details of relatives of 372 epileptics. Of 5533 relatives they found 700 epileptics, 535 alcoholics, 350 cases of feeblemindedness, 169 of insanity and 141 of migraine; 2427 members were without nervous disorders.

TURNER's (1911) earlier figures taken from 676 cases of epilepsy, revealed the fact that the commonest predisposing cause of epilepsy is ancestral epilepsy. In a further series of 214 cases, in which parental alcoholism as a predisposing influence was especially inquired into, the same conclusions were arrived at, viz, that ancestral alcoholism was a relatively minor factor compared with ancestral epilepsy in the causation of the disease. TURNER found no hereditary cause in 350 cases or 49 % (first series), in 106 cases or 49.5 % (second series), he found epilepsy in 250 cases or 37.2 % (first series) 81 or 37.8 % (second series); he found alcoholism in 21 cases or 3.1 % (first series), 15 cases or 7 % (second series). There are many cases in TURNER's material where nothing is known of heredity. Therefore the percentage of the known causes is also low.

COLLINS (1913) in 177 cases of epilepsy obtained an ancestral history of defects in 101 cases or 57%. The defect was alcoholism in the parents or the grandparent in 57 cases or 32.2 % of the total. Of the 320 males of a second series of cases, parental alcoholism is recorded in 72 instances or 22 % ; in 10 cases both parents were drunkards; of the 100 females alcoholism occurs in the parents in 28 cases. Of the 72 cases of parental alcoholism the heredity is paternal only in 54 cases and in the 28 females it is paternal only in 22 cases.

FAIRBANKS (1914) in a critical study of 175 cases of epileptic children found in only 12 instances traces of convulsive attacks in the ancestors or in other members of the family. He found many cases of trauma during pregnancy and birth. He does not mention parental alcoholism. THOM (1915) studied 157 cases of hereditary epilepsy, each presenting 1 or more of the following five mental defects: epilepsy, alcoholism, insanity, feeblemindedness and migraine. He found in 58 of these hereditary cases alcoholism of the ascendants (in 42 cases of the father, in 9 cases of the mother, in 4 cases of maternal grandfather and in 3 cases of paternal grandfather). The number of times that alcoholism is found alone is 23 i.e. 14.6 %. In 95 % of the cases where alcoholism, migraine or feeblemindedness was the defective influence, the heredity was direct. Epilepsy associated with alcohol and epilepsy with migraine were the two commonest combinations of the hereditary tracts.

Of 204 sufferers from epilepsy in JÖDICKE's (1914) material, there are 108, i.e. 50.4 % with direct and indirect hereditary transmission: of these 44 times i.e. 31.9 % by alcoholism (32 times or 39.5 % in males and 12 times or 21 % in females).

The figures of others are as follows: (cit. JÖDICKE) SIEBOLD 18 %, BIRO 14 %, FINCKH 25.7 %, WOLFENSTEIN 43.5 %.

MEDOW (1914) finds in 12 cases of epilepsy 3 cases of alcoholism in one of the parents accompanied by traces of other psychical defects

VOGT (1910) as psychiatrical consulting adviser to a polyclinic for children was struck by the fact that among youthful psychopaths with serious alcoholic ascendants, there were so many instances of epilepsy or epileptically disposed children. These were nearly always the offspring of non-Jewish families. (page 22) As a special observation, the following instance deserves to be mentioned: VOGT (1910) describes a healthy woman who had children by three different fathers. One was an illegitimate child of a healthy peasant lad, another was also an illegitimate and epileptic child of a tramp and drunkard and five children were conceived in her marriage with a steady man. Only the second child of the seven was ailing. BIANCHI (1911, cit. STÜBER) found in 511 epileptics who attended the psychiatric polyclinic at Naples in the course of 10 years, that 30 % of the cases could be attributed to alcoholic heredity. According to FLOOD and COLLINS 1913 (cit. STÜBER) there is still no proof that parental alcoholism causes epilepsy in the children. BOLTEN found in 121 cases of epilepsy potus of the genitor as the only hereditary tract in 8 cases, tuberculosis in the family 7 times and in 36 % of the cases he found marked heredity.

STUCHLIK (1918) scrutinized the history of about 12600 patients who were admitted into the psychiatric clinic at Zürich in the years 1870/1913 and found among them 341 sufferers from epilepsy. Of 176 epileptic patients, there were 89 cases of alcoholic heredity i.e. 30.2 % (there must therefore be some patients with hereditary transmission of more than one relative), of these 55 times in case of father, 10 times mother, 6 times in paternal grandfather, once in grandmother, 6 times in uncles and aunts, 6 times in maternal grandfather, grandmother once, aunts and uncles 4 times. In 58 % of epileptic patients with alcoholism in the ascending line there was no other illness in the ascendancy.

In the case of married alcoholics, STUCHLIK found from the material of the psychiatrical clinic at Zürich, that of 50 children there are only 28 (56 %) healthy, 5 (10 %) are epileptic. He is of the opinion that alcohol is a very frequent cause of epilepsy (page 69).

WYRSCH (1921) found in Unterwalden 57 epileptics i.e. 1.85 per 1000 of the population. (AMMANN estimated for the whole of Switzerland the number of epileptics at 5 per 1000). The aetiology of this material of WYRSCH's is, 22.8 % heredity, 24.6 % parental alcoholism and 7.35 % traumatism. The polyclinics of Zürich were attended in the years 1913—1919 (resp. 1920) by 418 epileptics. The aetiology of 165 cases is: 13.5 % heredity, 15.9 % alcoholism, 15.3 % trauma.

BOVEN (1918) reports on 48 epileptics of both sexes in the asylum at Cery Switzerland 30 cases of heredity from paternal alcoholism i.e. about 60 %.

O. MARBURG (1919) finds with 150 chronic epileptics, 60 males and 90 females, 41 cases of hereditary transmission, of which alcoholism 5 times. He accepts 10—19 % alcoholic aetiology of parents.

MUSKENS (1924) found that in 1000 male and 1000 female epileptic patients, quite a third of the cases showed epilepsy (also migraine and in pregnancy) in·the families (ascending line direct and indirect and descending line). MUSKENS found insanity in about 15 % of the cases. MUSKENS says that alcoholism in the parents and grandparents is certainly a disposing influence for epilepsy in children. In the above material he found 48 cases of alcoholic heredity of parents and grandparents in 911 males and 63 similar cases in 900 females, thus in 6 % of the material.

From the information contained in the literature it appears therefore that the significance of the use of alcohol by the parents as a cause of epilepsy in children is really very great. Many investigations especially about the use of alcohol in the ascending line of epileptics have been made, but fewer about epilepsy in the descending line of alcoholics.

There are, especially among later investigators, some who doubt the significance of parental alcoholism for the origin of epilepsy in the children.

REDLICH (1924) observes that it is often possible to prove without any doubt parental alcoholism in the ascending line of young epileptics, but proof to the contrary is lacking, that is to say from the corresponding percentages in non-epileptic children. REDLICH finds in the material of his own practice where epilepsy in general is less prevalent, that alcohol plays no role with the parents of epileptic patients.

HAUPTMANN (1917, p. 209) also observes that in his material of a Research-department for nervous diseases during the great war, parental alcoholism played a very small role, at least as sole cause.

RÜDIN (1923) when looking the first time through his material, did not find a great percentage of sufferers from epilepsy among children of chronic alcoholics. Neither did WAUSCHKUHN, whose results of an examination of RÜDIN's material were communicated by SNELL (1921). BUMKE (1924) also agrees with RÜDIN. GAUPP (1925) likewise observes that the injurious effects of the use of alcohol by parents on the children has not yet been made clear.

The significance of parental alcoholism is still shown in the remarks made by VOGT (1910) that especially the early appearance of serious cases of epilepsy is not seldom found in children of drinkers (see also page 25).

RÜDIN's material of the Research Institute for Psychiatry at München was scrutinized by SNELL (1921). SNELL grouped his material in the same manner as KOLLER and DIEM (page 43) and those of KALB. He finds that alcoholism with epileptics is more often an hereditary factor (25.9 %) than with mental diseases (20.9 %) and with healthy people (21.3%) and much oftener than with general paralysis (14 %). Especially parental alcoholism is considerably higher than in the three other groups. WAGNER-JAUREGG (1928) points out, that SNELL finds in 352 cases of epilepsy 18.9 % hereditary transmission with alcoholism and only 3.4 % with epilepsy and concludes that parental alcoholism takes an important part in the aetiology of epilepsy. (Also E. MÜLLER, p. 23).

The results of the investigations by GUSCHMER (1916) pupil of RÜDIN, in which he found among parents of 54 epileptics 16 times alcoholism, herewith correspond. He found only seven times alcoholism among the 90 fathers of the cousins.

SNELL is uncertain either of the significance of alcoholic heredity as a germ injury or that for instance a hereditary influence at one time produces epilepsy and another time intemperance.

The information given by SNELL on the basis of investigations of WAUSCHKUHN made at the genealogical section of the Research Institution at München ,that chronic alcoholics have not always epileptic children is noteworthy (see also RÜDIN page 35). The descendants of alcoholics who were about 30 years of age, were examined. In the case of paternal alcoholism there is apparently some other combining influence in epileptic families which results in epilepsy in children. Moreover we would refer to divergent results of other authors.(table 3).

Of recent date investigations we may mention those of KÜFFNER (1927), GANTER (1927), NOTKIN (1928), WEISE (1928), GERUM (1928), OSTMANN (1928) and KÜENZI (1929). KÜFFNER (1927) compiled the following statistics of the material of an Institution for epileptics in Saxony. Of 900 epileptic women 12.3 % have in the direct ascending line or in side line epilepsy, 11.4 % psychoses and nervousness. 103 patients had hereditary antecedents of intemperance of parents or of grandparents, or if doubtful cases are included 124 patients, i.e. in 11 % or 14 % of the cases. 47 of these patients have not only parental alcoholism in the ascending line but also some psychical abnormalities. If these 47 cases are left out there remains only 6 % of the cases with alcoholism of the parents as sole hereditary factor.

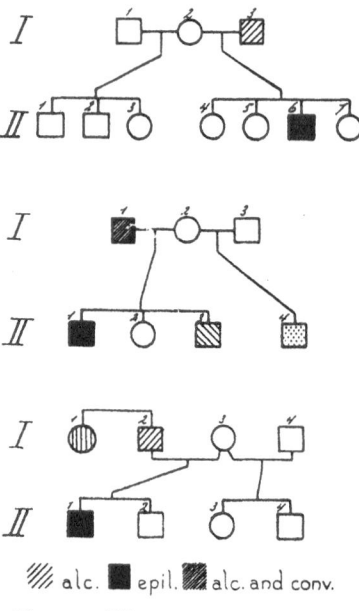

%% alc. ■ epil. %% alc. and conv.

N imbec. ::: bodily weak |||| bad temp

Fig. 1.

Pedigrees. (From GANTER, N. 19—21).

For 1100 male sufferers from epilepsy KÜFFNER found similar figures viz epilepsy in the ascendancy in 12.7 % of the cases, psychosis etc. in 13.8 % of the cases and alcoholism alone in 6 % of the cases.

GANTER (1927) examined in East Prussia the heredity in the ascending line of 503 sufferers from epilepsy. Of 106 of these patients there was an incomplete anamnesis and there were 104 cases of organic epilepsy; with 102 patients there were hereditary antecedants, 104 patients were without hereditary antecedants. Of the 102 patients there were hereditary antecedants of epilepsy 35 times (parents, uncles, and aunts), of epilepsy in brothers and sisters 18 times, of insanity 10 times, of abuse of alcohol by father 23 times, of nervousness 15 times, and of imbecility in the father once.

GANTER reports some cases (see Fig. 1) where one of the parents had been married twice. If then one of the parents was alcoholic, epilepsy was found in the offspring of the intemperate parent; similar cases were also reported by VOGT (1910, see page 23) and HOLITSCHER (cit. by GANTER). In the 106 cases with insufficient anamnesis there were in 20.7 % of the cases hereditary antecedants of epilepsy and in 36.7 % of the cases of alcoholism. This last percentage is very high according to GANTER: the interrogating physician will have been too hasty in filling in alcoholism. When GANTER put all the different groups of his material together he found in 503 sufferers from epilepsy 66 times hereditary antecedants of alcoholism i.e. in 13.1 % of the cases. (However, the 3 groups when checking GANTER's figures do not comprise 503 but 233 cases (102 + 25 + 106 = 233; 23 + 4 + 39 = 66). The percentage of 13.1 named by GANTER is incorrect.)

NOTKIN (1928) an American worker says that ancestral alcoholism has been emphasized by many investigators. He gives a detailed review of the literature in which it is shown that investigators found alcoholism in the ascending line in 20—30 % of the cases. NOTKIN found in his own material in 39 cases, 4 cases of maternal alcoholism; and 5 cases of paternal alcoholism; in 2 cases both father and mother were alcoholics; in one case paternal and maternal grandfathers; finally in one case paternal grandfather, the father and a brother were all alcoholics. There are thus 13 cases in which there is a direct ancestral alcoholism giving 32.5 % of the total number of cases and 48.1 percent of the number with known heredity. The frequency is slightly higher on the paternal side. Although NOTKIN is aware of the doubt of some investigators as to the reliability of the frequency of alcoholism in the ascending line of epileptic patients, he found in his own small material a high percentage. NOTKIN observes that he has met with the same difficulties in obtaining reliable family records which have been mentioned by other investigators (DÉJÉRINE p. 20).

GÜNTHER WEISE (1928) a pupil of KEHRER's found with genuine epilepsy besides other factors as hereditary antecedants also potus.

GERUM (1928) made a thorough investigation of the heredity of epilepsy in the material of the hospital for mental and nervous diseases in Frankfort a. M. in the years 1921—1926. He made exhaustive enquiries in the families. This is therefore an important investigation.

Epilepsy is in Frankfort a rare illness. GERUM found rather a large number of cures and a great number of cases of a mild character. He is of the opinion that epilepsy does not contribute towards degeneration. GERUM's special object was to learn to define the whole of the epileptic symptomes better with the aid of investigations of heredity. He combines in a first group the cases of epilepsy with direct, similar heredity (thus parents and grandparents and again epilepsy). GERUM has 12 of such cases (6 fathers, 6 mothers and moreover one case of the grandfather of the father). In this group GERUM investigated alcoholism as well. In 4 of the 12 families there was potus of one of the parents, of two very slight. It is clear that these selective cases do not form a complete idea of the significance of alcoholism for the aetiology of epilepsy.

GERUM examined also the children of his patients. The figures are small, 23 children of these epileptic families without potus do not differ from healthy families. The picture is not so favourable (infantile mortality, imbecility) of 35 children of these epileptic families with potus. According to GERUM, the material of the children with ancestral alcoholism is markedly inferior to that of epileptic families without potus. In a second group GERUM combines 18 cases of indirect similar heredity (8 times brothers and sisters, 6 times cousins). Also in this material there is a small hereditary antecedant of alcoholism.

A third group comprises 42 cases without epileptic antecedants; GERUM calls them singular cases; although without antecedants of epilepsy it still includes the antecedants of insanity and nervous disease, also of parental alcoholism. In 62 % of the cases there was alcohol in the anamnesis that is to say, the patient himself is alcoholic or the family is addicted to drink. The significance of alcohol in this 3rd group is much greater than in both of the preceeding groups, which depends on the grouping. GERUM compares in the 3rd group the epileptic patients in families where alcohol is misused with those in families where alcohol is not misused and found the percentage about the same (the same result as GERUM found with the other groups). This result does not say much as to the significance of the abuse of alcohol for the aetiology of epilepsy because the numbers are so small. One might expect the number of epileptic children in alcoholic families to be larger than in as large a number of sober families.

GERUM in his conclusions on this basis, observes that alcohol might not be ascribed the capacity of producing genuine epilepsy. This far reaching conclusions, that te made on the basis of a small amount of human material and with his mind fixed on the simple Mendelian figures for segregation, may certainly not to be accepted for such a complicated subject as epilepsy.

His conclusion is also that the investigations covering offspring in cases of epilepsy may only be made in such cases where alcohol plays an unimportant part. The important investigations of GERUM which have little bearing on the question of parental alcoholism, point out the necessity of family investigations concerning alcoholism. (see p. 61).

OSTMANN (1928) examined the extracts in the Lunatic Asylum at Schleswig. From 1900 till 1925, 520 patients were admitted for epilepsy. Of 218 patients he reports hereditary antecedants, of which there were 71 cases of alcoholism in the ascending line i.e. 33 %.

In the material of KÜENZI (1929) with 31 men and 3 women, who suffered from epilepsy and alcoholism at the same time, there were 90 births and 4 still births among the males and 13 births with the females. Before the end of the 2nd year there died 16.1 % of the children of the male group and 7.7 % of the female group, together 15 %; 17 % of the children died before reaching their 20th year. Among the grown up children 2 suffer from epilepsy (2.9 %), 3 from psychoses, 4 from alcoholism and 2 from imbecility. KÜENZI finds about the same figure in the group epilepsy only. In the ascendancy we find 14 cases of alcoholics out of 51 males and 8 cases of alcoholics out of 44 females epileptics i.e. 23.2 %. Of epileptics who at the same time were alcoholics the alcoholic heredity was 58.9 %.

In table 3 the results of some investigations are summarised. The percentage of epileptic patients among whom alcoholism in the ascending line is present, varies very much (tab. 3 column 2). There are several reasons for this. Abuse of alcohol has been accepted by different investigators more or less easily. The material varies also. If alcoholism of relatives of the patients is traced by consulting old histories of diseases (historiae morbi) one will in general obtain less reliable results than when the investigator pursues the abuse of alcohol in the families by questioning the patients present at a certain moment and by paying visits. Furthermore there is a difference in the

TABLE 3. ALCOHOL ABUSE AMONG THE RELATIVES OF SUFFERERS FROM EPILEPSY

Author	Alcoholism in the ascendency of epileptic patients [1]		Alcoholism only in the ascendency of epileptic patients		Epilepsy in the descendency of alcoholics	
	%	N. [2]	%	N.	%	N.
MOREAU (1854)	19.35	124				
LANCERAUX (1879) . .					25	410
„ „ . .					33	241
A. VOISIN (1883) . . .	12.6	95				
J. VOISIN (1897) . . .	31	299				
MARTIN (1879)	70	83			33	
DÉJÉRINE (1889) . . .	51.6	350				
FÉRÉ (1890)	38.3	308 m.				
„ „	45.4	286 f.				
BOURNÉVILLE (1901) .	36.5 [4]	2554 [3]				
„ „ .	3.1					
„ „ .	1.5					
ECHEVERRIA (1881) . .			18.2 m.	572 [5]		
„ „ . .			16.2 f.			
„ „ . .	17.2 [6]				20.25	
DEMME (1890)	30	98				
LEGRAIN (1895)					25	215
„ „ . . .					20 [7]	481
GRIFFITH (1911) . . .	5.2	154				
O. BINSWANGER (1899) .	22	121	6.5	121		

[1] Some authors distinguish in the ascendency the direct heredity (parents, grandparents) and the collateral heredity (sisters and brothers, uncles and aunts).

[2] We only mention the number of patients, of which family data have been obtained. Some authors mention also the total number of patients.

[3] Cf. p. 20 Sufferers from epilepsy, hysterics and idiocy. The total number of admissions, patients without a family anamnesis are included.

[4] Alcoholism of the father, of the mother of both parents.

[5] Alcoholic epileptics.   [6] Among ordinary epileptics.

[7] Epilepsy and hysterics; after correction; without correction 17.2 %.

TABLE 3 (*continued*)

Author	Alcoholism in the ascendency of epileptic patients [1]		Alcoholism only in the ascendency of epileptic patients		Epilepsy in the descendency of alcoholics	
	%	N. [2]	%	N.	%	N.
GALLE (1899) [3]	2	607 m.				
SULLIVAN (1900) . . .					4.1	219
KRAEPELIN (1913) . . .	18.2	303 m.				
„ „ . .	19.2	104 f.				
„ „ . .	21	267 [4]				
VOLLAND	29	24	12.5	24		
LUI [5]					12	
MUNSON (1911)	50	78 [6]				
E. MÜLLER (1910) . . .	34	503				
SICHEL-SIOLI (1910) [7] .	16	726				
GRENIER [8]					24	195
NEUMANN [8]	23.7				16.4	
STÜBER (1921)	33					
TURNER (1911) [9] . . .	3.1	676				
„ „ . . .	7	214				
COLLINS (1913)	32.2	177				
„ „ . .	22	320 m.				
„ „ . .	28	100 f.				
FAIRBANKS (1914) [10] .		175				
THOM (1915)	37	157	14.6	157		
MEDOW (1914)	25	12				
BIANCHI [10]	30	511				
FLOOD and COLLINS [11] .						

[1] See page 32.   [2] See page 32.   [3] Cf. page 22.
[4] Younger than 20 yrs.   [5] Cit. by H. VOGT.
[6] Traumatic epilepsy.   [7] Sufferers from epilepsy, hysterics and imbecillity.   [8] Cit. by E. MÜLLER.
[9] no heredity known 50 %.
[10] Parental alcoholism not mentioned.
[11] Cit., by STÜBER and p. 25.

TABLE 3 (*continued*)

Author	Alcoholism in the ascendency of epileptic patients [1]		Alcoholism only in the ascendency of epileptic patients		Epilepsy in the descendency of alcoholics	
	%	N. [2]	%	N.	%	N.
BOLTEN			6.4	121		
STUCHLIK (1915) . . .	30.2	176	17.6	176	10	50
WYRSCH (1921)	24.6	57				
„ „ . . .	15.9	165				
BOVEN (1918)	60	48				
MARBURG (1919) . . .	10—18	150				
MUSKENS (1924) . . .	5.2	911 m.				
„ „ . . .	7	900 f.				
SNELL (1921)	25.9				[3]	
GUSCHMER (1926) . .	30	54				
KÜFFNER (1927) . . .	12.3	900 f.				
„ „ . . .	11 (14)	124	6	124		
„ „ . . .	13	1100 m.	6	1100 m.		
GANTER (1927)	22.5	102 [4]				
„ „	36.7	106				
NOTKIN (1928)	32.5	39				
GERUM (1928)	62 [5]	42 [6]				
OSTMANN (1928)	33	218				
KÜENZI (1929)	23.2	95			2.9	

figures of column 2, because some investigators of those patients forming the material, leave out those of whom there are no or insufficient family records, or also leave out where there are no hereditary antecedants. There are also differences of opinion as to the conception of heredity. Some investigators include also patients with signs of degeneration. There is also a difference, owing to the fact that

[1] See page 30.   [2] See page 30.   [3] Cf. p. 27.
[4] All with hereditary transmission.
[5] Without heredity by epilepsy.
[6] Alcoholism in ascendancy or of the patient himself.

under heredity sometimes only the heredity by the parents and grandparents, in other cases by all relatives is understood. Further, investigations concerning patients in institutions may not simply be placed in the same category as those concerning patients at large (those who attend polyclinics). The country or district where investigations are made is also perhaps of importance with a view to the great difference in the percentage of epileptic patients in different territories. Yet it would be very wrong to wholly deny the demonstrative value on the grounds of the objections which may be brought forward to many of these statistics. After all, there is too much conformity in all these statistics to allow this. We may positively assume that among the ascendants of epileptics there is a frequency of alcoholics in 20—30 % of the cases.

Investigations as to the presence of epileptics in the offspring (descendants) of alcoholics are very much less numerous. A percentage of 15-20% is found (6th column, table 3). We have already mentioned the observation of RÜDIN (see also WAUSCHKUHN) that he in his material among the children of alcoholics found very few epileptics. An important finding by GERUM is that the children of epileptics with potus in the ascending line show greater inferiority than those of epileptics without potus in the ascending line. How alcohol in the ascending line has acted, either as pure heredity or as germ poison (see p. 18) is difficult to determine. From column 4 of table 3, it may be seen how frequently — only a few investigators have reported here on — alcoholism appears as the only cause in the ascending line of epileptics (cf. page 75).

In the future, importance will mainly be attached to those investigations where the investigator himself knows his material, and where he has obtained the family records by his own questioning and visits and when he does not limit his questioning to alcoholism alone. From short descriptions of all or a number of the cases (as the old French clinical investigators did) the reader will be able to see how the investigations have been made and which likewise enables him to judge the cases. It is also of importance that the investigator collects control material, thus examining healthy people in the ascending and in the descending line. And when investigating the descendency of alcoholists it is necessary to trace their ascendency. It is only possible to judge the significance of the alcoholism of the parents for deviations in the descendants, if one knows as well as possible the genotype of the parents.

3. Feeblemindedness, Imbecility and Idiocy

As in the aetiology of epilepsy alcoholism of parents has an important part, as it also has for feeblemindedness. BOURNEVILLE examined 1000 cases; of 829 cases there was alcoholism of one of the parents, 620 times i.e. 75 %; drunkenness of father at conception is reported 57 times. J. VOISIN (1897) reports that alcoholism appears most frequently in the statistics of idiocy and that drunkenness also causes idiocy in the descendants. ECHEVERRIA (1881 p. 491) observes that of idiocy the direct cause is parental alcoholism in contrast with epilepsy and other nervous disorders, which would appear together with alcoholism alternately in the families of alcoholics. (p. 21). ECHEVERRIA will here no doubt be especially thinking of serious affections of the brain (hydrocephalus e.g.).

LORRAIN (1871, cit. by KRAEPELIN) also believes that the causes of dystrophic infantilism are especially injuries of the germ by diseases of the parents: lues, tuberculosis, alcoholism and perhaps malaria and pellagra as well. (p. 75).

ECHEVERRIA himself finds parental alcoholism in 35 % of 211 cases of simple and epileptic congenital idiocy. Three of these idiots were conceived while their respective fathers displayed manifest signs of alcohol intoxication (p. 58). 27 or 12 % of 225 alcoholic epileptic patients with hereditary antecedants of epilepsy, insanity or intemperance had idiot brothers or sisters. ECHEVERRIA reports further that LANGDON DOWN believes that intemperance in the parents produces only 2 % of idiocy in offspring, whilst F. BEACH finds parental intemperance in 31.6 % out of 430 patients and KERLIN in 38 cases out of 100 idiot children.

DEMME (1890) finds in his material of the children-hospital at Berne, that of 61 feebleminded, imbeciles and idiots of 1—4 years, there were 33 from families where the father was inebriate i.e. 54 % of the cases. Seven of these children, which just comprised the imbeciles and idiots, the mother was also potator. In a second group of 53 similar children there were 29 cases of hereditary antecedants of parental intemperance i.e. 55 %. Nothing is said in how far these children themselves also received alcohol.

LEGRAIN (1895) found 322 feebleminded children in 814 cases of children of alcoholics i.e. 39.5 %.

BEZZOLA (1901) informs us of his experience as Asylum doctor and doctor of an establishment for feebleminded children, that on one side there is a frequency of heavy drinking of parents of the feebleminded and on the other side there is much feeblemindedness of children in the descending line of drinkers.

SICHEL (1910) found among the patients of the lunatic asylum where parental alcoholism was reported, 10.4 % suffering from imbecility and idiocy. SCHLESINGER (1907, 1926) examined 138 pupils of schools for feeblemindedness from 128 families. He found 49.2 % with psychoneurotic heredity (21.6 % seriously insane) and 30 % alcoholism of parents. SCHLESINGER reports in 1926 that in his material more than the half consists of mentally deficient children from drinking families, and he refers to the significance of heredity and of environment.

The poor vitality of offspring of drinkers according to SCHLESINGER is conspicious. It is distinctly less then that of other pupils. Two thirds of the number show distinct degeneration and half of them had shown convulsive dispositions in first year. PILCZ (1907 ref. RÜDIN 1908) found with imbecility, alcoholic psychoses and epileptical mental disorders, alcoholism in the ascending line as most important influence. BAYERTHAL (1910) found as doctor of a school for the feebleminded in Worms 59 times in 64 children i.e. 92% of the cases hereditary antecedents in the form of nervous and psychical disorders, mostly in the parents. In the same material Bayerthal found in 53 % of the cases alcoholism of the father.

The divergent findings of ELDERTON and PEARSON (1911) we have already discussed (p. 12). We pointed out that PEARSON himself ascribes them to the exceptional manner in which his material is compiled. H. VOGT (1910) found among jouthful psychopaths very many children of drinkers, but he also thinks that the children attending the schools for the feebleminded emanate from families with limited mental power.

STROHMAYER (1910), physician of an educational home for children, is of the opinion that in feeblemindedness, alcoholism of the parents plays a greater role than heredity.

MEDOW (1914) found in the first place that with congenital

feebleminded persons serious injuries to the germ play an important part. Of 15 of the cases there were 4 referred to as cases of hard chronic alcoholism of one of the parents.

ROSENBERG (1914) has in his material (p. 61) 27 cases of imbecility; in 10 of these parents or grandparents were drinkers.

In 42.6 % of the cases KRAEPELIN (1915 IV, 2311) found hereditary transmission by the parents to be the cause of imbecillity and idiocy and 22 % of these cases through alcoholism.

ELIASSOW (1915) pursued the material of a school for backward children in Königsbergen in Prussia in another manner than PEARSON. He investigated the history of families of which at least two children attended or had attended the school. As a medical man he visited the families himself. He had data of more than 50 families, 73 children of which were attending the school during the investigations. ELIASSOW gives the pedigree of all families. In this instance the method of working was correct but still incomplete; the intellect of the family was only investigated in a small degree and we must remember, that it is selective material.

ELIASSOW found alcoholism in the family anamnesis of 43 children, i.e. 58.9%. In his material alcoholism is by far the strongest hereditary influence. He found imbecility in the ascending line only twice, the same with insanity, and with epilepsy four times. The infantile mortality is very great, 30.9 % (tab. 2, p. 14). Only such persons where abuse of alcohol was clearly found (repeated drunkenness, degeneration of character and neglect of family) have been annotated. Of the 73 children, 23 or 31.5 % had inebriate fathers.

E. DE VRIES (1917) found in an asylum 22% of the cases of idiocy from parental alcoholism. HERDERSCHEE (1925) informs us that in 2663 children attending schools for backward children, there was parental alcoholism to the extent of 14%, alcoholism of the grandparents occurs in 43% of the cases.

WEINBERG (1918) opposes the idea of a strong propagation on the part of mental defectives. In any case this only applies to those in the married state. The frequency of marriages among mental defectives is, however, small. The mental defectives according to WEINBERG would become extinct if they were not continually formed anew. WEINBERG thinks that alcohol in the first place plays an important role.

REITER and OSTHOFF (1921) found of 250 pupils of a school for backward children alcoholism of one or both parents 54 times — 21.6 %. The whole hereditary transmission for alcohol in the ascendency is 23.6 %.

Of 235 children from families where one or more children attend this school for backward children, and of which one of the parents is imbecile there are, according to the investigation of REITER and OSTHOFF (1921), 192 i.e. 50 % weakminded. Of 133 children, however, of which one of the parents is moreover a drinker there are 99 i.e. 74.4% weakminded. The ratio with children of drinkers is therefore less favourable. In the families which are taxed with alcoholism and weakmindedness only 9.2 % cases are found, where no other weakminded brothers and sisters are; in the families which are only taxed with weakmindedness this percentage is much higher viz. 26.2 %.

With 63 children at the same school one of the parents is weakminded, the other a drinker; of these 63 children there are 49 weakminded thus 77.8 %. With 70 children of this school one of the parents is healthy, the other is weakminded and drinker at the same time Of these 70 children there are 50 weakminded i.e. 71.4%. According to these figures there may be besides the disposition for weakmindedness also a toxic influence of alcohol.

This conclusion is not forcible here: one must know the genotype of the children.

GANTER (1927) found in his patients suffering from imbecility and idiocy 56 cases of hereditary transmission, 61 cases with no hereditary transmission, 28 cases where family anamnesis was insufficient and 148 cases where the deficiency was caused through organic defects. In the 56 patients of the first group there was 18 times alcoholic hereditary transmission, 11 times feeblemindedness, 4 times insanity and 9 times abnormalities in character. Furthermore there were six cases with dual transmission, whereof the transmission from father's side was 5 times alcoholism. In the group with incomplete family data, the hereditary factors were: alcoholism, feeblemindedness and abnormalities of character. LOKAY (1929) found with parents of 82 imbeciles, 25 cases of alcoholism i.e. 30 %, of which 6 times imbecility. LOKAY estimates after correction the number of alcoholics among the parents at 15.8 %. BRUGGER found 14.8 %.

Among fathers alone LOKAY finds 32.9%. In the feebleminded, where there was alcoholism in the ascending line, there were many short-comings in character (SCHLESINGER).

According to BUMKE (1924) it is certain that the exogenic cause of idiocy arising from injuries to the germ through alcohol (quicksilver and lead) and syphilis, is more frequent than the endogenic.

RÜDIN finds epilepsy and imbecility more frequently occurring together among brothers and sisters than f.i. imbecility, and manic depressive psychosis. This can indicate germ poisoning by alcoholism of the parents.

From table no. 4 we see that the different authors find different percentages of hereditary transmission. Our conclusions are the same as for table 3 (page 31).

TAB. 4. ALCOHOLISM AMONG THE RELATIVES OF SUFFERERS FROM IMBECILITY AND IDIOCY

a. Alcoholism in the ascendancy

Author	N.	N. of cases.	%
BOURNEVILLE	829	620	75
ECHEVERRIA 1881	211		35
Beach	430		31.6
KERLIN	100		38
DEMME 1890	61	33	54
„ 1890	53	29	55
BAYERTAL 1910	64		53
MEDOW 1914	15	4	27
KRAEPELIN 1915			22 [1]
KING [2]			11.3 [1]
SCHULTZE [2]			15 [1]
KÖNIG [2]			15 [1]
FREDGOLD [2]			46.5 [1]
GUILLAUME [2]			41 [1]
SCHLESINGER [2] [3]			30 [1]

[1] Parents.   [2] Cit. Kraepelin.
[3] Investigation of children of schools for backward children.

Author	N.	N. of cases.	%
LEUBUSCHER [1] [2]			20 [3]
POTPESCHNIGG [1] [2]			33 [3]
LEY [1] [2]			42.4 [4]
KOLLER [1]			30 [3]
IRELAND [1]	235	76	32.3 [3]
KRAYATSCH [1]	433	40	9.2 [4]
„		8	1.9 [5]
ELIASSOW [2] 1915	73	43	59
E. DE VRIES			22
REITER and OSTHOFF 1921	250	54	21.6 [3]
			23.6 [6]
HERDERSCHEE	2663		14
			43 [7]
SCHMID-MONNARD [8]			11
HENNEBERG [8]			11.5
CASSEL [8]			29
ZIEHEN [8]			20.3
HILLENBERG [8]			2.5
SCHLESINGER 1926			50
GANTER (1927)	56 [9]	18	32
LOKAY 1929	82	23	30 [10]

b. *Imbecility in the descendancy of alcoholics*

Author	N.	N. of cases	%
LANGDOWN DOWN			2
LEGRAIN 1895	814	322	39.5
DEMME 1890 (Cf. p. 000)	57	47	

[1] Cit. Kraepelin.
[2] Investigation of children of schools for backward children.   [3] Parents
[4] The father.   [5] The mother.   [6] Entire hereditary transmission.
[7] Alcoholism with one of the grand parents.
[8] Cit. Reiter and Osthoff.   [9] Patients with hereditary transmission.
[10] After correction 15.8 % among the parents.

4. Malformations

The occurrence of idiocy, epilepsy and malformations in families has been written about very often and as a cause of these defects parental alcoholism has also been mentioned. VOGT (1910) states that he knows of several pedigrees where very serious forms of psychical degeneration, epilepsy and idiocy and serious malformations, still born and such like occur. (cf. RÜDIN, p. 40).

LAITINEN mentions that in his material he also met deformed children.

DUVAL and MULON (1912) report that the cause of malformations is due to parental alcoholism and even ordinary drunkenness at time of conception (page 58).

LANCERAUX (1879) found in the descending line of drinkers, inebriates, feeblemindedness and epilepsy, also malformations. The malformations meant here are, malformations of the brain, causing hydrocephalus and porencephaly. Further he mentions individuals, badly developed in body, small of stature with asymmetry of the skull. MAGNUS HUSS (cited by LEGENDRE 1912) also ascribes congenital weakness to alcoholic heredity. (Infantilism, LASÈGUE, BAER). LANCERAUX points out the decrease of length of body of children of tuberculous alcoholics (small stature in wine districts).

Parental alcoholism is responsible for the increase of the number of persons rejected for military service according to BAER and DEMME (1890). DEMME found of 47 cases of hydrocephalus, 23 cases of hereditary transmission through parental alcoholism (17 times by the father, 4 times by the mother and twice by both).

ARRIVÉE (1899) found congenital bodily weaknesses in the group of alcoholism of the parents in 3.85 %, in that with tuberculosis in 1.2 % and in the indefined group in 0.75 % of the cases. (See also page 10).

Bodily defects, stigmata, deformed skull, asymmetry, dental malformations, deafness, paralyses, pathological curvature of the spine were found by LEGRAIN (1895) in 29 out of 215 alcoholic families.

ROGER (1912) also says that racial degeneration appears in stigmata of body, decrease of the length of body and nervous diseases, epilepsy or hysterics and insanity and he refers to the statistics of DEMME in this respect. DEMME's (1890) statistics are certainly very important (cf. page 67). Of 57 children of 10 families of alcoholics, there were only 10 normal, 25 died young, 5 are bodily bad developed and 4 deformed. Of 61 children of 10 parents, who do not drink there were 50 normal, 5 died young, 2 with congenital deformities. E. SCHWALBE (1906 page 179, 1911 page 574) is of the opinion that it is certain that syphilis and alcoholism of the parents mean signify serious injuries to the fetus, often causing death. It is however not certain that these diseases can be indicated as a cause of definite types of malformations (see also page 81, STOCKARD).

ARRIVÉE (1899) found in 1506 accouchments, 17 times twins, i.e. 11.3 per thousand. Of the 17 cases there are 9 in the group for parental alcoholism, which comprises 383 cases i.e. 23.5 per thousand. ARRIVÉE reminds us of the opinion of TOURNIER that twin pregnancy is to be considered as a form of hereditary malformation. Also in LUNDBORG's table (p. 60) many malformations appear as the expression of alcoholic transmission of parents.

Where there are different symptoms of inferiority in children, such as feeblemindedness, epilepsy and malformations in the family of an alcoholic one is especially included to think of blastophtorical effects of alcohol. (page 72). The occurrence of malformations in tuberculous families is attributed by FÉRÉ (1894, page 371) to the effects of the tuberculous toxin in the developing embryo (p. 1).

5. Insanity and Neuropathy

Among the children of alcoholics MARTIN found epileptics, idiots and imbeciles, sufferers from insanity and hysterics.

French clinicians attach much importance to the use of alcohol of the parents as a cause of insanity. JOFFROY (1895) says that parental alcoholism is most frequently found in the heredity of the insane and this is perhaps the most significant.

KOLLER (1895) one of FOREL's pupils has studied the material of patients of the years 1881—1892 in the lunatic Asylum at Burgholzli. Of the 1850 patients, there are 49 % with antecedents of insanity, 20.5 % of alcoholism and 19 % of psychopathy. The patients with alcoholic heredity are especially sufferers from alcoholic psychoses and epilepsy and congenital mental deficiencies (imbeciles and

idiots). Of the 30 patients suffering from alcoholpsychoses there were
40.4 % with alcoholic heredity (see page 47).

KOLLER investigated the ascendency of a similar number (370) of
healthy persons and patients. She found 76.8 % hereditary trans-
missions with patients (for the whole material the hereditary transmission was 78.2 %) and 59 % with healthy people. These are remark-
ably high figures; perhaps among the healthy there are a number of
special characters, psychopaths with hereditary transmission which
should really be separated from the healthy.

The 59 % hereditary transmission of healthy persons covers 28 %
direct transmission; the 76.8 % heredity of patients comprises 57 %
direct heredity. The difference between healthy persons and patients
in respect to the direct heredity is considerable (1 : 2). As to the
direct heredity of the healthy persons, the percentage of the total of
persons with hereditary transmission (218), of insane inheritance is
10 % of nervous diseases 11 % and 14.2 % (31) of alcoholism. Concerning the direct heredity of patients, the percentage of hereditary
insanity is 25 % for the total number of those with hereditary
transmission (284) of nervous diseases 7.4 % and 19 % (54) of alcoholism. There were 45 cases of indirect inheritance. Of 370 healthy
people there were 31 (8.3 %) with alcohol parental heredity and of an
equally large number of patients there were 45 (12 %) which had
the same form of inheritance.

LEGRAIN (1895) found among 761 children of drinking parents 145
times insanity i.e. 19 %.

ANTON (1901) found with 5000 admittances at the psychiatrical and
neurological clinic at Halle 460 times alcoholism of the parents i.e. in
10 % of the cases.

DIEM (1905) who made similar investigations to KOLLER's found
with healthy men 64 % of the cases to be of hereditary transmission
(in the ascending line) and with women 69.5 %.

Through alcoholism of parents, mentally deficients are somewhat
more taxed than healthy persons. There are in KOLLER and DIEM's
material lunatics with parental alcoholic heredity: men in 23.6 %,
36.4 % and 27.6% of 713, 748 and 595 cases respectively and women
17.4%, 28.0% and 17.9 % of 734, 522 and 596 cases respectively.
In DIEM's material the direct inheritance is of parental alcoholism

with healthy persons in 11.5 % and with mental deficients in 13—
21 % of the cases.

The method of investigation made by KOLLER (1895) and DIEM
(1905) is of special importance. They compared the hereditary
transmission of lunatics and of healthy persons and distinguished
in the cases of inheritance the number from insanity, from psychopathy and from alcoholism. In this the high figures for healthy persons are marked and surprising.

The investigations teach us that when making medical statistical
investigations about parental alcoholism, we must always make
control investigations with healthy people. With experimental investigations this has already become the custom. (See also page 77).

TIGGES (1907, page 893) reports from German institutions 41.4 %
hereditary transmission, of which 8.3 % from alcoholism in the
ascending line.

GEELVINK (1907) found among 100 female chronic alcoholics treated in the Lunatic Asylum during the last four years, 12 imbeciles, 13
with hysterics, 8 with epilepsy, 4 psychopaths and 3 women who
became alcoholics in the climacteric, together 40 % congenitally deficient persons. Among 800 male admittances during the same period
with chronic alcoholism there were 32.2 % congenital deficients.
Among the remaining female chronic alcoholics there were still 4
with hereditary insanity and 9 times alcoholism of one of the
parents. With the remaining 600 male alcoholics these figures were
8.6 % and 4.6 %. The influence of environment is shown in the
fact that 40 % of the female alcoholics as prostitutes, waitresses and
public women were connected with the liquor trade through their
profession.

From this publication of GEELVINK's it again appears that the
notion of hereditary transmission must be defined more sharply.
There must be discrimination between heredity in respect to parents
and that of other members of family. Further congenital deficiency,
imbecillity for instance is not simply hereditary transmission. In
the case of epilepsy the use of alcohol by the patient himself has
also been wrongly referred to as transmission. Other investigators
also include bodily and nervous stigmatism in the notion of hereditary transmission (page 31).

Further the investigations made by SICHEL (1910) in 1907 and

1908 of people voluntarily taken up in the Lunatic Asylum at Frankfort are important. Of 2523 patients there were 449 with alcoholic heredity (342 males and 107 females) i.e. in 17.7 % of the cases, 304 times with nervous diseases, 335 times with insanity and 1440 times there was no such inheritance, or it was unknown.

Of these figures there were some cases of persons having been admitted twice: the number of patients with hereditary antecedents of alcoholism, i.e. abuse of alcoholism by the parents (in 248 cases) or by close relatives (60 cases) amounted to 308 cases(225 males and 83 females). Among these patients there were especially chronic alcoholics (123), further sufferers from imbecility and idiocy (32), from hysterics (23), from epilepsy (47) and alcoholic psychoses (53, principally delirium tremens) and from other forms of insanity (62).

The hereditary transmission by alcoholism with the patients of the Lunatic Asylums refers namely to alcoholics and sufferers from the different alcoholic psychoses (in all 176 of 308 cases) and in a less degree persons suffering from other forms of insanity (62 of 308 cases). In other material SICHEL found of 714 admittances 93 cases of parental alcoholism i.e. 13 %.

Finally I would point out the association of alcoholism of the parents and dementia praecox, which various writers refer to. SICHEL finds among patients with alcoholism in the ascending line 14.3 % suffering from dementia praecox.

JELLIFFE (1911) e.g. finds that three elements have been most marked in the ancestry of dementia praecox patients, viz. dementia praecox itself, alcohol and abnormal personality. Alcoholic parents have according to JELLIFFE's experience, been mostly responsible for hebephrenics.

BERZE points out that different cases of chronic alcoholism and alcoholic psychoses could be included as similar heredity with dementia praecox. Alcoholism is very often an accessory to dementia praecox and not seldom the expression of hebephrenics.

In his extensive material on heredity of patients suffering from dementia praecox RÜDIN finds (1916) in the group of families with sufferers from this psychosis, where one of the parents was addicted to drink, the percentage of dementia praecox patients greater than in families where alcohol was not consumed by either of the parents. The same with HUTTER (1926).

RÜDIN's results would point out that alcoholism of one of the parents favours the condition for dementia praecox.

BERZE and JELLIFFE see in alcoholism of one of the parents in those cases often the symptoms of an abnormal character even of dementia praecox, to which alcoholism in its turn has been attributed. In the instances named by JELLIFFE (1911), alcoholism has been a symptom of severe neurasthenia or even dementia praecox at a more advanced age, and to which it in its turn has contributed and established a vicious circle which has left its impress in heredity.

POLISCH (1927a) finds among 60 chronic alcoholics (not delirium tremens) 64 % with abnormal dispositions. POLISCH does not mean cases where psychosis arose later, but psychopaths (epileptoid-irritable, over-sensitive, epilepsy, unbalanced). POLISCH thinks that such psychopathical deficiency and not a psychotical disposition is the basis of chronic alcoholism (contra STÖCKER). Therefore chronic alcoholics are not latent sufferers from dementia praecox.

Of various nervous diseases, hereditary transmission through alcoholism of the parents is named.

DEMME (1890) found in 61 cases of chorea minor 19 times alcoholism of the parents i.e. in 31 %. FRETS (1929) finds in five families suffering from RECKLINGHAUSEN's disease, several members of families with alcoholism and with tuberculosis.

In table 5 we see some examples of the percentage of alcoholic heredity of relatives, mostly the parents (see also page 61).

6. Alcoholism and Abuse of Alcohol by the Parents

The difference between heredity of use of alcohol and germ injury through use of alcohol of the parents is perhaps shown best, if we try to determine the significance of the occurrence of alcoholism in the ascendency of alcoholists.

We can imagine alcoholism i.e. the desire for drinking alcoholic beverages and for satisfying it to be hereditary. ESQUIROL (1838) already points out that the fatal disposition to drunkenness is sometimes hereditary. There is sometimes, he says, a marked inclination which induces certain individuals to make an excessive use of fermented beverages.

KROON (1924) reports on a case where the heredity of drunkenness

TABLE 5. ALCOHOLISM AMONG THE RELATIVES OF SUFFERERS FROM
INSANITY

a. Alcoholism in the ascendancy

Author	N.	N. of cases	%
KOLLER	1850		20.5 [1]
id.	30 [2]		40.4
id.	284		19
ANTON 1901	5000		10
KOLLER and DIEM 1905	713 [3]		23.6
id. . . .	748 [3]		36.4
id. . . .	595 [3]		27.6
id. . . .	734 [4]		17.4
id. . . .	522 [4]		28.0
id. . . .	596 [4]		17.9
TIGGES 1907			8.3
SICHEL 1910	714	93	13
id. 1910	2532	449	17.7

b. Insanity in the descendancy of alcoholics

Author.	N. of children	N. of cases	%
LEGRAIN 1890	761	145	19

is quite clear. With members of this family intemperance is either
very marked or is completely absent; there are no cases of moderate
drinking. In this family members of the first generation, the male as
well as the female were not at all given to drink. Several sons, thus
belonging to the 2nd. generation are intemperate whilst the daughters are wholly free of intemperance. Among the sons of these daughters, thus in the 3rd generation, cases of intemperance again make
their appearance, whilst the daughters do not show this characteristic.
On the grounds of a thorough investigation of this family, which

---

[1] There are among them especially sufferers from alcoholpsychoses.
[2] Alcoholpsychoses.   [3] Males.   [4] Females.

comprises 140 members of which 16 drunkards, Prof. KROON comes to the conclusion that we have to do with a case of sex-limited heredity (MORGAN, WOODS). Intemperance would be dominant with the male and recessive with the female.

We can imagine that the use of alcohol injures the germcells and that through this mentally and physically inferior individuals, epileptics, imbeciles, idiots, malformed and insane are born. That in this manner persons are born with the inclination for alcoholic beverages, is only conceivable in so far that mental deficients have a weak will. Different investigators (e.g. MINOR 1910) points out the difficulty in getting an impression as to how the inclination to use some artificially prepared chemical product or other can be inherited (cf. idiosyncrasy; p. 113).

ECHEVERRIA (1881, page 495) referring to histories of the descent of 115 individuals, who have exhibited symptoms of alcoholism, notices that the number of children amounts to 476 and that drinking instincts have manifested themselves in 205 of them. LEGRAIN (1889) studied the admittances of alcoholics at Lunatic Àsylums and found of 119 alcoholics, 63 times alcoholism in the ascendency, after correction he arrives at 63 cases of alcohol heredity out of 102 individuals, i.e. in two thirds of the cases. In 1895 he found with 215 drinkers 108 times alcoholism in the descendency i.e. in 49 % of the cases; or of 467 children there are 197 alcoholics i.e. 42 %.

LANCERAUX finds with 813 admittances of alcoholists in the hospitals, 174 times alcoholic heredity i.e. 21 %.

ANTON (1901) finds with 460 cases of alcohol psychoses and neuroses 250 times intemperance of the parents i.e. in 54 % of the cases. DODGE (cit. ANTON) finds with 379 drunkards in an asylum 180 times alcoholic heredity (47 %). SOLLIER (cit. ANTON) finds in 350 families with chronic alcoholism 40 % hereditary transmission and of this 106 cases of parental alcoholism i.e. 30 %. Prof. HITZIG says ANTON, on the basis of his clinical experience, was of the opinion that the children of alcoholics were more disposed towards nervous diseases than the children of nervous and mentally deficient parents (page 44). HEYMANS and WIERSMA (1906) as a result of their investigations of the heredity of a great number of characteristics, including intemperance, are of the opinion that these characters are more or less subject to heredity. SICHEL (1910) finds among 2532 patients, 822 cases of alcoholism. Of these 822 cases there are 224 instances of hereditary transmission through potatorium of parents or close relations i.e. 27 % of the cases. PILCZ (cit. V. WLASSAK 1929) finds in 60.9 % of the cases of alcoholism, parental alcoholism.

RYBAKOW (1906) investigated the material of the polyclinic of the Psychiatrical Clinic in Moscow. He questioned in all 600 alcoholics who applied for medical advice, about the question alcoholism and nervous diseases of parents, grandparents, brothers and sisters and uncles and aunts. Alcoholism in the ascendency is found by RYBA-KOW in 87 % of the cases; 21% of the cases exhibited nervous and mental diseases among near relations. RYKABOW concludes that alcoholics just as other morbid persons are strongly disposed to bring similar children into the world. To become a drinker, say RYBAKOW and others, one must be in the first place born as such. With the very great percentage of the hereditary transmission in RYBAKOW's material one must also bear in mind the influence of environment (page 73).

Alcoholism of the parents (the father) is found in alcoholics in a very high percentage by MINOR (1911) and PREISIG and AMADIAN (1918). MINOR investigated the heredity and the conditions of life of the patients (total 9760) while attending a polyclinic for alcoholism in Moscow. For the year 1907 he finds that in 88 % of the 9760 cases, many relatives, members of the families of alcoholics were also alcoholics. Of 1812 alcoholics there were 1378 intemperate fathers, 1414 brothers and 1186 uncles on the father's side, 385 on the grandfathers side etc. After these investigations, the result of which struck MINOR very forcibly, he made other investigations for 1908. Of 158 patients there are 113 alcoholic brothers, 103 fathers, 58 uncles on the fathers side, 55 on the mothers side, etc. MINOR who knows the profession and residence of his patients, refers to the great influence of environment (maladie des camarades, FÉRÉ).

Conforming findings were reported by PREISIG and AMADIAN (1918) pupils of MAHAIM of the Asylum at Cery in Lausanne. They observed 100 cured alcoholics from the material of the Blue Cross Society in Switzerland. The duration for the abuse of alcohol was four years at least, the mean duration 15.5 years. The period of abstinence was at least 5 years, the mean duration 19 years and was on an average at the ages of 22—37 years. Most of the patients drank land wine, at least 1 Litre per day. Others more (15 individuals 5 litres, some 6—10 litres). The average age when abusive drinking was commenced was 23 years. The authors examined their own material, the persons and the conditions of living. The physical value of the persons examined was good in their youth, 80 % were fit for military service. Also in later years there was no indication of abnormal morbidity. All these people, especially those who were past sixty were strong and well preserved for their age. Very few psychical deviations were noticeable.

PREISIG and AMADIAN find for all their 100 cases, hereditary transmission, of which there is direct heredity in 86 cases. In 65 cases the heredity is alcoholism (65 %), in 14 cases abnormalities of character, 'in 4 cases insanity and 8 times suicide. There was direct heredity from fathers side in 80 cases, from mothers side in 6 cases and there were three cases of collateral heredity (brothers and sisters). The heredity on fathers side (80 cases) was for instance 62 times alcoholism. These are very high figures. Alcoholism as direct heredity with normal individuals is found by DIEM in 11.5 %, of the cases, with insane people in 21—25 % of the cases.

PREISIG and AMADIAN do report, it is true, on the descendancy of the cured alcoholics, but as they did not examine the descendents personally, these data do not come into consideration for them for forming an opinion. This is certainly a great pity, as observations of the children of the cured alcoholics among whom there would be many adults would just be of great importance.

STUCHLIK (1915) finds among 50 children of married alcoholics only 4 (8 %) alcoholics (or suffering from another disease).

MALEIKA (1926) finds in the ascendency of the sufferers from alcoholism which made its appearance again after the great war 22 % hereditary transmission, mostly in the form of alcohol abuse of father. OSTMANN (1927) likewise finds in the ascendancy of sufferers from alcohol psychoses (576 men and 59 women) in the Lunatic Asylum in Schleswig in the years 1899—1926, 22 % hereditary transmission through alcoholism of parents or grandparents. KÜNZLER (1930), see tab. 6.

POLISCH (1927a) finds that nearly half of the fathers (33 of 69) of sufferers from delirium tremens made an abusive use of alcohol. POLISCH sees here especially the influence of environment (page 73).

TABLE 6. ALCOHOLISM AMONG THE RELATIVES OF ALCOHOLICS

Author	N.	N. of cases	%
LEGRAIN 1895	119	63	60
LANCERAUX	813	174	21
ANTON (1901)	460 [1])	250	54
DODGE (cit. ANTON)	379	180	47
SOLLIER (—)	350	106	30
SICHEL 1910	822	224	27
RYBAKOW 1906	600		87
MINOR (1911)	9760		88
ROSENBERG 1914			45
PREISIG and AMADIAN (1918) .	100		65
OSTMANN (1927)	635 [1])		22
POLISCH (1927)	69	33	50
POLISCH (1927).	33 [2])		50
KÜNZLER (1930)	303	114	38

b. Alcoholics in the descendancy of alcoholics

Author	N. of alcoholics	N. of children	N. of alcoh. children	%
ECHEVERRIA 1881 . .	115	476	205	43
LEGRAIN 1895	215	467	197	42
STUCHLIK 1915 . . .		50	4	8
POLISCH 1927	58	123	1	0.8

Among the drinking fathers there are two cases of delirium tremens; with 22 brothers and sisters addicted to alcohol (total 304) there was one case of delirium tremens. More than half of 33 female sufferers from delirium had fathers or mothers who drank. Other forms of hereditary transmission are not to be found in POLISCH's material.

---

[1]) Alcoholic psychoses.   [2]) Females.

He has excluded the cases of feeblemindedness in the ascendancy (page 70).

OSTMANN (1927, page 250) finds of 40 sufferers from delirium only four without any hereditary transmission. Of these 4 patients one was suffering from chronic lead poisoning, one had undergone a trauma, a third one was physically very weak and a fourth was physically ill. Of hereditary transmission OSTMANN mentions 56 times alcoholism of the father, once of the family, once of the grandfather and once of the brothers and sisters; once the father was insane, three times the mother, 4 times the father was suffering from nervous disease or had an abnormal character, there are 6 times hereditary transmission without further details, two illegitimate children, 2 imbeciles, 4 persons with numerous signs of bodily degeneration. One sees that OSTMANN takes a broad view of hereditary transmission (p. 31).

The investigations of OSTMANN and POLISCH cannot be compared. POLISCH works on selective material; he chose cases without hereditary transmission in order to trace the nett significance of parental alcoholism in the descendency (page 73). NÄCKE (1912) is of the opinion that with delirium tremens there is nearly always predisposition. DEMME (1889) likewise thinks so.

BOSS (1929) among 1057 (909 males, 456 females) admittances of alcohol patients in the mental hospital in Zurich in the years 1910 to 1927, among the alcoholics, who besides, before their inebriation, showed some mental defect and who almost without exception had some psychopaths and insanes in their ascendancy, in 45 % of the cases, finds that the father was an alcoholic.

He finds the same percentage for alcoholics only.

He also finds the same percentages with alcoholics alone and complicated alcoholics for the alcoholism of other relatives (brothers, mother and sisters). This is a remarkable result, which points to the significance of alcoholism as an influence of environment rather than of heredity. In so far as alcoholism belongs to the characteristics of the "famille neuropathique" we shall expect to find alcoholism oftener in the ascendancy of psychopaths than in those of healthy people.

BOSS finds among alcoholics in the alcohol trade a smaller number of psychopaths and persons with hereditary transmission than in the rest of his material (p. 72); the proportion is 1 : 3. 95 married alcoholics in the alcohol trade whose wives were not heavy drinkers, have 233 children. The first five years 196 children survived (see tab. 2). All these children are physically and mentally sound except those in two families. In one family of three children all three are physically backward, but mentally sound; in a second family there are three healthy children and one epileptic child. Boss remarks that for further understanding family investigations are necessary. From the material of the consultation bureau for alcoholism he has taken 4 families where there is much alcoholism in the ascendancy, but no other form of mental inferiority. In these families there is no increasing inferiority among the children and grandchildren (p. 64). The children, however, are often still young and the families are very insufficiently known; moreover the data are for the greater part procured by laymen.

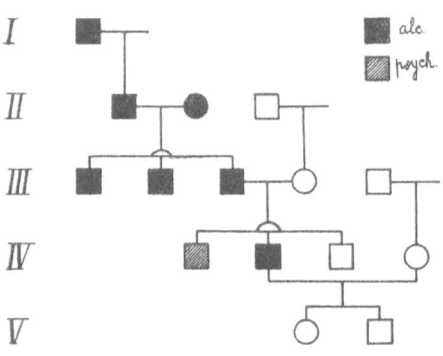

FIG. 2. Pedigree (Ped. E, from Boss, 1929) The children V 1 and V 2 are in a rather good condition, V 2 is bodily weak and nervous. In four generations the father was an alcoholic. There is very little known of other parents.

In table 6 we see again very divergent figures. With normal individuals DIEM finds in 11.5 % of the cases alcoholism as direct heredity.

If we compare the tables 3—6 about the occurrence of alcoholism in the ascendancy of sufferers from epilepsy, imbecility, idiocy, insanity and alcoholism and about the occurrence of these diseases in the descendancy of alcoholics, we cannot determine either which of the diseases is more frequent with parental alcoholism, owing to the divergent percentages in every list. The percentages for imbecility and idiocy are somewhat higher than for epilepsy and insanity. The figures for alcoholism are the highest because tradition is of importance here.

When judging these results we must take into consideration how often imbecility and idiocy, epilepsy and insanity occur in the as- and descendancy of normal people.

7. Tuberculosis

The association of alcoholism of the parents with tuberculosis in the children is very complex.

If as a consequence of the abuse of alcohol by the father a reduction of the income of the family is brought about, the general conditions of life, feeding and living become worse, and by this the disposition of the children for tuberculosis becomes enhanced.

Furthermore the father who drinks is more exposed to infection with tuberculosis through frequenting public houses (la phthisie se prend sur le zinc, HAYEM) and the children in their turn are exposed to the danger of contagion. Chronic alcoholism of the father has also an injurious effect on all organs of the body, also on the germ-cells (blastophthory), so that weak children with also reduced power of resistance against tuberculosis are born. Children of alcoholic parents contract tuberculosis more readily than children of temperate parents (tab. 7 page 56). These are phaenotypical phenomena.

Many experiments have been made from which it has been proved that the use of alcohol reduced the resisting power against infection (KERN, 1910).

Further tuberculosis, besides alcoholism and other defects, are considered as a component of the "famille neuropathique" (FÉRÉ, RIETEMA 1904). For so far as this connection exists, tuberculosis in the children is genotypically defined. Finally, with regard to the descendancy of tuberculous patients, the toxin of the tuberculous bacil is a germ poison (page 1) and for this reason children of sufferers from tuberculosis will have a lesser resistance in very many respects, thus also against the inclination to use alcohol. In the descendancy of tuberculosis patients one can on these grounds expect more alcoholics.

LEGRAIN (1895) found among 814 children of potators 55 times tuberculosis i.e. 6.77 %.

IMBAULT (1901 cit. STOCKARD) found tuberculosis to be about as common among children of alcoholic parents as among those of uberculous parents.

ROSENBERG (1913) found an unfavourable influence of parental alcoholism on the tuberculosis in the children and a still worse influence from the alcohol itself.

From table 7 we see the significance of parental alcoholism for tuberculosis in the children.

TABLE 7. (After G. VON BUNGE)

Alcohol consumption of the father	N. of cases	Tuberculosis of the father % of cases	Tuberculosis of the children % of cases	Nervous and mental diseases of the father % of cases	Nervous and mental diseases of the children % of cases
Not regular [1]	430	4.9	11.6	2.6	9.3
regular but not much [2] . .	480	5.8	11.7	3.1	14.3
steady drinker [3]	231	7.4	21.7	4.3	22.2
heavy drinker	167	12.6	29.3	4.8	27.5

8. The capacity of the mother to feed her child

In different publications since 1899 VON BUNGE deals with the results of his investigations about the ability of the mother to feed her children. He finds that the ability to do so is on the decrease and indicates as the cause the use of alcohol by the parents. In the course of 10 years VON BUNGE sent out to the doctors lists of questions and found that of 2401 cases, 883 mothers were able to give their children the breast, and 1518 were not able to do so. Of the latter number 450 women were not able to feed their children although their respective mothers had been able to do so.

VON BUNGE investigated the occurrence of tuberculosis, insanity and nervous disease, caries and alcoholism (tab. 7).

In the group of 450 women, who could not feed their children

---

[1] Drinks occasionally.

[2] Daily consumption less than 2 L. beer or less than 1 L. wine or a herewith corresponding quantity of other alcoholic drinks.

[3] daily consumption 2 L. beer or one L. wine or more.

themselves, although their own mothers had been able to do so, VON BUNGE finds that in 40 % of 338 cases the father was potator (in the sense of hard abusive drinking) and in 33 % was a hard drinker. In the group for women, where both mother and daughter had been able to feed their children, the father in 1.8 % of 605 cases was a potator and in 6.8 % a hard drinker. In the group of 545 women, where mother and daughter both were unable to feed their children, these percentages were 14.6 and 14.3.

It would appear that in the first group where the mother was and the daughter was not able to feed the children that the abuse of alcohol by the father is highly significant. In the 3rd group where both mother and daughter were unable to feed heredity plays a part. In these families there is also more insanity and nervous disease and more tuberculosis.

AGNES BLUHM (1908) finds among 39 daughters of alcoholics only 14, thus 36 %, who could not feed their children. V. WLASSAK (1929) points out that the material is small and there is an absence of control observations so that it therefore cannot be taken as a contradiction of the results of V. BUNGE.

It is of importance to note also, and to which BLUHM refers to herself, that BLUHM investigated the descendancy of alcoholics in respect to the feeding capacity of daughters, whilst V. BUNGE investigated the ascendancy of mothers not feeding their children (page 35; also p. 72).

9. Parental Alcoholism and Crime

DUGDALE (1877) in his studies of criminals finds that 42.5 % of the total number of criminals are of intemperate families while 39 % are habitual drunkards. For DUGDALE it is more than probable that the common causes of both crime and intemperance are notably sexual excess and insane ancestry. BAER, giving figures for the prisoners in Germany, states that 24 % are suffering from the hereditary effects of parental alcoholism. These criminals were at the time that they committed the crime occasional drinkers or alcoholics. (BAER, p. 48).

From the report of ANTON (1901) I cite that BENDA finds with 500 criminals hereditary transmission of parental alcoholism in 30 % of the cases, MARRO 46 % with 507 criminals and TAWNOWSKA 54 % of the cases with 150 prostitutes.

JÖRGER (1905) finds in the Zero family among 240 adults, 20 criminals. Crime is not very prominent here. See also LEGRAIN (page 68)

Of 199 criminals observed by HARTMANN (1905) in the prison at Zürich there are 35.2 % with alcoholic heredity and 32.7 % criminal heredity. These figures according to another calculation are 29.6 and 19.1 %. DIEM found for healthy persons, comparable with the last named figures, 17.7 % and 10.4 %. With criminals there is therefore a considerably higher alcoholic transmission than with healthy persons. Parental alcoholism is in the case of criminals one of the most important hereditary influences. The direct heredity (i.e. through parents) amounted to 26.1 % with these 199 criminals (23.1 % through the fathers) .Of the 199 criminals themselves there were 63 or 29.4 % alcoholics. Among the habitual criminals there are roughly twice as many drinkers as among occasional criminals. The former have also almost twice as large an alcohol heredity and two and a half times direct heredity. Of the criminals with alcohol heredity a much greater number are alcoholics themselves than of criminals, who have no alcoholic antecedents or who have some other hereditary influence. BAER (cit. HARTMANN) finds with 17.418 Prussian prisoners 22.5 % with direct alcohol heredity and with 4087 Bavarian 34.6%. The percentages found by other authors are among others 16.1 %, 25 %, 30 %, 46 %, 69 %.

HARTMANN has made investigations with 214 criminals from the day of their birth i.e. about the significance of acute alcoholism of the progenitors similar to those made by BEZZOLA for feebleminded persons (page 59) and finds his results confirmed. (cf. also V. WLASSAK, 1929).

10. Acute Parental Alcoholism

We have seen that alcohol consumed by man is taken up into the blood and the tissues (page 3) and if we therefore trace the phenomena of the use of alcohol to the quantity of alcohol in the blood, we can imagine that an acute and serious alcoholic intoxication (drunkenness) during coitus leads to a defective new individual, either an imbecile, idiot or an epileptic.

There are some reports of observations of defective children whose parents admitted drunkenness during copulation (ESQUIROL, FÉRÉ 1884, 1890, A. VOISIN 1883, DÉJÉRINE 1886, TOULOUSE 1896 and BOURNEVILLE). Of the present standpoint regarding heredity, one would like to know the genotype of the parents (thus the occurrence of diseases, epilepsy, insanity, imbecillity in the ascendancy). The drunken father may also be a chronic alcoholic (O. BINSWANGER 1899).

WOODS (1913) reports on children, conceived during drunkenness of the father and who became epileptic; the fathers were usually nondrinking persons and all the other children were healthy (p. 28). E. MÜLLER (1910) reports similar cases.

BEZZOLA (1901) investigated with the aid of statistics the significance of acute parental alcoholism for the occurrence of feeblemindedness in children. His material was 8196 cases of imbecillity and idiocy occurring according to the official census of 1897 for children in the canton Berne, born between 1880 and 1890.

BEZZOLA fixed the number of births, in each month of the year of these feebleminded children and compared this with the number of children of the general birth statistics and he then found that with months of heavy drinking among the population, carneval time, vintagging, are corresponding months in which in general fewer children were born, yet there were more feebleminded individuals among these than in other months. The differences are not very great and there are still other influences. It is clear that it is difficult to conclude from these data that there is some connection here between the drunkenness of conception and the imbecility of the children. Of the statisticians PEARSON (1910) sharply criticized such a conclusion. MÜLLER (1910) made similar investigations in respect to epilepsy. The material he had at his disposal was small, namely 847 cases. He also arrived at a result that in such times when alcohol is principally consumed the production of abnormal children occurs. Similar investigations were also made by HARTMANN (1905) with a small number of 214 criminals, with the same results (p. 58). NÄCKE (1908, 1912) pointed out the difficulties to obtain anything definite on this point (lit.). HOPPE (1910) admits these difficulties yet he describes in a historic review the great value of the proofs. O. HERTWIG (1913) considers it very improbable that acute alcoholism

TABLE 8. (From LUNDBORG).

Classification of the Groups.	Number of Families	Number of Children.	Mean number of Children in each Family	Died before 5 years.		Healthy Persons over 15 years.		Statements of defect.		Defective Persons.		Defective to a high degree.	
				Number	percent	Number	In percent of the survivors over 5 years.	Number	percent	Number	percent	Number	percent
I. Parents with no hereditary transmission	30	148	4,9	27	18,2	85	70,3	23	15,5	22	14,9	2	1,4
II. Tuberculosis in one or in both parents	14	52	3,7	19	36,5	22	66,7	8	15,4	8	15,4	1	1,9
III. Excessive use of alcohol in one or in both parents	37	213	5,8	56	26,3	69	44,0	84	39,4	70	32,9	26	12,2
IV. Parents are related, besides in many cases other hereditary transmission elements	57	392	6,9	116	29,6	129	46,7	134	34,2	106	27,5	44	11,2
V. One or more hereditary transmission elements in the parents	102	586	5,8	114	19,5	251	53,1	203	34,6	166	28,0	61	10,4
I—V Together	240	1391	5,8	332	23,9	556	52,5	452	32,5	372	26,7	134	9,6

would give rise to the said deviations; he is, however, convinced that chronic alcoholism has an injurious effect on posterity.

11. Family Investigations

Just as besides or above the statistical treatment of a subject much importance is attached for medical consideration to a detailed account of individual cases, so in the treatises on alcohol detailed information of well observed families or groups of population is of great value.

JÖRGER (1905), the Physician in chief of a Hospital for Mental Diseases in Switzerland, describes the Zero family, of which he himself knew three generations. Of the 310 persons in 5 generations and during more than a century, records are given. Vagabondism, alcoholism, crime, immorality, feeblemindedness and insanity are the features of this family, alcoholism being predominant.

The injurious effect of the use of alcohol by the parents, as a germ poison is to be clearly seen in the family, says JÖRGER. In a family of which both parents are drinkers, the progeny is exceptionally bad. There is hereditary inferiority in the family and the outward circumstances are also unfavourable, yet the alcoholics have the worst progeny. On the other hand all improvements in the family are accompanied by a lesser use of alcohol. JÖRGER also described the Markus family.

Investigations made by DUGDALE (1875) in the JUKE family in which are many criminals are also very well known (page 57).

ROSENBERG (1914) went through the family records of 100 families of a small village in the 19th century ("die Amberger"). He finds the average age of drinkers lower than with moderate drinking people. The infantile mortality up to the age of 20 years is greater with children of heavy drinkers than with moderate drinkers. Among the children of moderates there are fewer drinkers than among those of drinkers. Here, therefore, is clearly a question of heredity. Of the population of this village observed by ROSENBERG, 45 % certainly emanate from drinkers, while of the adult men only 30 % descend from drinkers. The results are exceptionally bad where the father and mother both drink. The influence on the children is stronger if the mother drinks than if the father drinks. PEARSON who also finds this, thinks he can ascribe this to neglect where the mother drinks. ROSENBERG says that the decided impression one gets when studying the tables of families, that a number of families are declining rapidly, unfortunately cannot be expressed in figures. Alcoholism occurs in certain families. 31 of the 103 families described by ROSENBERG include:

- 41 % of all persons,
- 40 % of all males above 20 years
- 80 % of all drinkers
- 56 % of all minors (large families)
- 56 % of all those supported
- 65 % of the whole amount of support
- 63 % of all feebleminded
- 46 % of all sufferers from tuberculosis and
- 37 % of all psychoses.

H. LUNDBORG (1914) now director of the State Institution for Heredity Research in Uppsala, has for many years been occupied with the population of a certain district in Sweden; he lived there from 1908—1912 and utilised all his time for studying the families. In his large book he describes the history of a farmer's family covering a century and a half; it covers 2200 persons, 377 families with 1909 children. He compares the data about these families with those of the whole Swedish population. In the larger family many cases of feeblemindedness, idiocy, insanity, psychoses, epilepsy are found. Also cases of alcoholism. Here, again, we are dealing with a family with its own constitution so that the conclusions may therefore not be generalised. (see also page 65).

In one group of the material studied there are 37 families where more or less serious alcoholism of one or both parents occurred (table 8). Further there was with these families no hereditary transmission. The families where alcoholism made its appearance after the birth of the children have not been included. The number of births in the group where parents are alcoholics is great, also the infantile death rate is great. In group I, where the parents are without hereditary transmission there are 15.5 % feebleminded persons, in the group III beforementioned, where one or both parents are alcoholic, there are 39.5 % (see table). Among these are, besides the insane, especially alcoholics and criminals. The number of healthy persons above 15

years is smaller than in any other group, viz. 44.5 %. Group I without hereditary transmission has the maximum number, being 70.3%
Cases of severe mental deficiency appear most in group III, in 12.2 %
of the cases; in group I in 1.4 % of the cases. LUNDBORG formulates
his opinion in this manner (page 493). It is to be regretted that we
have so far only an insufficient knowledge of the germ injurious factors. This is true, but in my opinion it is at least very probable that
alcohol plays an important part in respect to the creation of pathological mutations (defects) with human beings and I believe that in
degenerate families this may arise more easily than in healthy ones.

We must admit the great value of these investigations, because
LUNDBORG studied his material for many years personally.

Of the family No. 136, described by the psychiatrist SCHWEIG-
HÖFER in 1926, the abuse of strong drink is specially characterised.
The observation covered 7 generations. The writer concerned himself
with this family for 30 years, examined and treated a large number
of the members of the family personally. It is not possible for the
writer to discriminate in this family between the influence of environment and predisposition. In every generation there are several
potators; there is some influence of environment through profession
(innkeepers). Degeneration in the sense of progressive inferiority in
the successive generations was not found by SCHWEIGHÖFER. Besides
cases of alcoholic psychoses, also dementia praecox and manic-
depressive psychosis occur. Of the children of inebriates neither the
occurrence of epilepsy nor of feeblemindedness is mentioned. Most of
the inebriates among the members of the family are cyclothym.

LÖWENSTEIN (1928) reports of a pedigree which comprises more
than 2300 persons and which covers 8 generations. In this family
there were 42 sufferers from dementia praecox, 14 from different
psychoses, 7 from dementia senilis, 1 from general paralysis and 1
from maniac depressive psychosis, further there were 101 psychopaths, 68 drinkers and 11 criminals; a remarkable fact being that
there were no cases of epilepsy. The condition of the progeny is unfavourable.

We must take it, in respect to the result of these few family investigations, that with different families, the susceptibility for the
injurous effects of alcohol varies. There are some alcohol proof
persons (cf. page 77). Secondly, so far there are very few cases of

epilepsy in the families of alcoholics. These results are preliminary and coincide with some results named in the statistics already discussed (p. 35).

The family investigations also prove in cases of parental alcoholism, the importance of disposition or heredity, of germ injuries and of environment and tradition.

LUNDBORG is of the opinion that the significance of germ injury can be established. In a number of families in his large material, the only hereditary influence is alcoholism of the parents.

ROSENBERG got the impression that the many drinking families observed by him in his material, show a decline in the successive generations. JÖRGER finds that the alcoholics in the families observed by him have the worst offspring and that where the abuse of alcohol is stopped there is a rapid improvement Finally SCHWEIGHÖFER did not find any degeneration in his family 136.

Family investigations will best go to show the importance of alcoholism.

12. The Influence of Parental Abuse of Alcohol in the Successive Generations

Under the name degeneration MOREL refers to "all the different unhealthy persons which appear to me to depart from a normal type which in itself contains the conditions indispensible for the continuation of the progress of the species." And the morbid changes in the successive generations are progressive: "the offspring of degenerates present types of progressive degeneration". Some of the degenerates show sterility and are therefore incapable of transmitting this type of degeneracy. Among the different causes of degeneration alcohol plays a great role. Many French writers accept the opinion of MOREL. Of the older English writers E. DARWIN also reports on the effect of alcoholism of the parents on succeeding generations. (See for lit. DEMME 1890). The early appearance in children of some abnormality of the parents (anteposition) is also considered as a sign of progressive degeneration (ESQUIROL).

As to the progressiveness of degeneration as a result of alcoholism, this has not been established in statistics and it will also be very difficult.

LEGRAIN (1895) finds in the second generation of his material more serious changes than in the first. He has the data of 98 alcoholic families at his disposal covering two generations and finds deviations 294 times, through alcoholism in the ascendancy. He especially finds imbecility and idiocy (in 54 families). In 42 of 96 families there are children which had convulsions and in 40 of 96 families epilepsy exists. In all cases, with the exception of eight, where the sick persons became adults, alcoholism has been established. Of 33 families cases of insanity are reported in 23 families. Seven families were observed covering three generations. The third generation comprises 17 children, all feebleminded (imbeciles, idiots), 2 are epileptic and 2 hysterical).

ROSENBERG'S (1914) opinion, that with drinkers and their offspring in contradistinction to sober people an inferiority of body, mind, morality and of social standing appears, I have already mentioned (page 61 "die Amberger im 19. Jahrhundert"). ROSENBERG from his material cannot reply to the question as to whether the beginning of the degeneration first appears as a result of alcoholism. In the KALLIKAK family which GODDARD (1912) investigated over 6 generations and where very much degeneration, imbecillity and crime was found, there is no clear progressivity of degeneration, nor in the Jukes family (comp. page 66).

LUNDBORG (1914) has tried to form an opinion for his extensive material as to the progressivity of degeneration. LUNDBORG as stated before, lived from 1908 till 1912 among a peasant population and from his experience with those alive and from annotations, which are to be found in the well kept population statistics of Sweden, he compiled a history covering a period of two centuries and a pedigree of one family in seven generations. The ancestor was born in 1721. Till 1909 the pedigree comprised 377 families, in all 2232 persons. There are 132 i.e. 35 percent consanguinous marriages, which is very high. The population of the province Blekinge, where this family lives, compared with the other parts of Sweden, is backward and has for ages been characterised by bad qualities. What do the data of this pedigree say now about degeneration i.e. in respect to progressive inferiority? Whilst the forefather held a very high position in social life, there is a progressive social decline in the succeeding generations. From the first to the fifth generation there was a very strong increase of the stock; afterwards in the sixth and seventh generation the increase is less (through facultative sterility). The death rate in the family is not greater than in the kingdom. Of the different diseases, tuberculosis occurs in 4.1 % of the members of the family. Psychical inferiority is present to the extent of 9.5 %; insanity in 2.28 %. In this race the percentage for insanity is greater than in the province Blekinge. Moral and social inferiority is shown in 15.2 % of the total number observed, and besides this there are 12.1 % chronic alcoholics. From other groups in the material also it is indicated that the number of feebleminded in the family is very high. Of the children one fourth of the total died before reaching the fifth year and one fourth are mentally deficient and one tenth of the total are highly deficient.

From this extensive material LUNDBORG has endeavoured to determine whether the deficiency increases. This is, however, not shown by the investigations and the material still falls short of the mark. In the generations I, II and VII the numbers are too small and in the generations V and VI there are many persons still too young. There are only the 3rd and 4th generations left (with 140 and 462 individuals) both of which are closed. We see from LUNDBORG's table that the number of deficient persons from these two generations practically correspond with each other. The number of generations even in this material is too small to determine in this manner if the degeneration increases or decreases in successive generations. It is therefore necessary to pursue such investigations from time to time after a number of years. LUNDBORG also thinks that this will be done.

The conception among medical men that the abuse of alcohol by the parents has a progressive influence on successive generations, is founded more on the observation of individual cases than on investigations instituted about this question.

13. The Progeny of Alcoholics

With the investigations of the significance of parental alcoholism we have pursued systematically the records of ancestors of sufferers from different diseases as to the occurrence of alcoholism and thereby have also mentioned the progeny of alcoholics. Now we should like to discuss here especially some investigations about the offspring of alcoholics i.e. the descending line. DUGDALE (1877) describes in "the

Jukes" the offspring of a drinker and vagabond in six or seven generations. Among 709 descendants there were 77 or 10.9 % criminals and 142 or 20 % received help. Prostitution was very extensive (50 %). We have here before us a description of the conditions of life of persons from a certain social circle (crime, alcoholism, prostitution, poverty and vagabondism).

MARTIN (1879) did not make investigations about the offspring of alcoholics, although it might appear so from the title of his publication.MARTIN (1879) described with epileptic patients the occurrence of parental alcoholism and then investigated in 60 such families, the conditions of life of the brothers and sisters. He also investigated the causes of death of the parents and grandparents (cf. page 19).

ECHEVERRIA (1881) referring to histories of the descent of 115 individuals, 68 males and 47 females, who have exhibited symptoms of alcoholism appearing in various forms, notices that the number of children in the respective families is 476, there being 282 males and 194 females. Of this total

     23 were stillborn (5 % cf. p. 15)
  107 died from convulsions in infancy (22.5 %)
     37 died from other maladies
     96 are epileptic (20 %)
     13 are congenital idiots (2.7 %)
     19 are psychotic
     61 show nervous diseases
     19 are scrofulous and crippled

and 79 adults between the ages of 20 and 47 are healthy. Drinking instincts have manifested themselves in 205 cases of the above descendants (43%), 28 of whom correspond to the healthy category (cf. page 49).

DEMME (1890) finds in 10 families with hereditary antecedants of alcoholism of one parent or both parents and moreover sometimes from former generations, a total of 57 children. In the first month 25 children died i.e. 44 % from weakness or convulsions, 6 children were idiots thus 10 %, 5 children showed symptoms of stunted growth, thus 8.7 %, 5 suffered from epilepsy since time of puberty, 5 children had malformations hydrocephalus, clubfeet and harelip. Of the 57 children from these drinking families there were only 10 i.e. 17.5 % normal physically and mentally strong.

DEMME made a parallel investigation with children of temperate families. There were 61 children. Four children died in the first few months from weakness and gastro-enteritis without convulsions, 2 children were feebleminded, 2 children suffered from chorea minor, one child had a harelip and another spina bifida, 50 children i.e. 82 % were normally disposed. The figures in the temperate group are more favourable than in the alcohol group. Of all these families one would like to know as exactly as possible the genotype that is to say the hereditary constitution. DEMME gives some information in this respect. In one of the drinking famillies there was a case of suicide of the mother and of the brother of the drinking father. In another case two brothers of the father were suffering from epilepsy. In a third family one of the brothers of the father was an alcoholic and died from delirium tremens. In a fourth family with three idiot children the brother of the father suffered from imbecility and epilepsy.

With regard to the ascendency of the ten sober families, DEMME states that in one family the grandfather became psychotic at the age of 52 and died of pneumonia the same year. In a second of these families a brother of the father committed suicide in an attack of depression.

LEGRAIN (1895) studied the offspring of alcoholics and his field covered 215 personal observations of drinkers. In all the 215 cases he had records of the first generation at his disposal, in 98 cases also of the 2nd generation and in 7 cases of the 3rd generation. The 215 drinkers in all forms showed moreover also other pathological phenomena. The 215 families comprised 508 individuals, in all of whom LEGRAIN reports physical and psychical deficiences. In 168 of the 215 families there were degenerative signs (nervousness, unbalance, feeblemindedness, imbecility, idiocy, immorality, crime); nervousness is reported by LEGRAIN 63 times, debility 88 times, moral deviations 32 times, serious criminals 13 times. Of the physical deviations (stigmata) LEGRAIN reports misformed skulls, asymmetries, dental malformations, deafness, paralysis and pathological spinal curvature; these he found in 29 families. LEGRAIN mentions the total number of children in his material which showed the diferent divergencies (cf. the different chapters about epilepsy, feeblemindedness, etc.

SICHEL (1910) observed the offspring of 130 of the 308 patients for whom alcoholism of the parents had been established, being of 2532 patients received in the years 1907 and 1908 at the Asylum at Frankfort on Main (cf. page 45). These children are therefore the grandchildren of alcoholics. Moreover there is a frequency of alcoholism among their parents (cf. p. 49). Of the 130 married patients there were 22 childless marriages (also no miscarriages), of 10 others no records were available. Of the 98 remaining patients, 205 children were reported as healthy, of 118 children nothing is known; there were 52 times miscarriages 20 children were stillborn, 75 died shortly after birth, 21 died from convulsions and 32 from infectious diseases. A total number of 200 children therefore died before, at birth or shortly after. Among the survivors we already named the 205 healthy children and the 118 children of whom health is unknown, there were finally 42 unhealthy and deficient children (feeblemindedness, nervousness, convulsions, etc.).

Among the 308 patients, crime is very great and the social position mostly unfavourable. The causes of feeblemindedness with these 565 children are certainly different. They are children of insane, neurotic and alcoholic persons,whose parents made an excessive use of alcohol. The high death rate of children and next to this the great number of feebleminded and unhealthy children among the surviving children is striking.

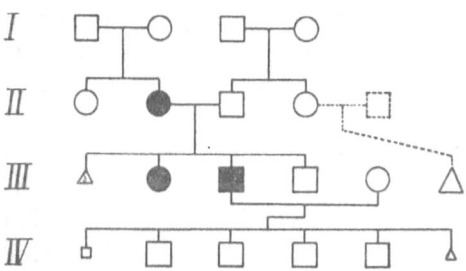

FIG. 3. Pedigree (from STUCHLIK, 1915) II 2 is alcoholic; II 4 has many illegitimed children; from II 2 three children died young, the 4th is alcoholic and a prostitute, the 5th is alcoholic and epileptic. III 5 has 6 children, the first died two weeks old of convulsions, the 2. and the 3. are passionate, the 5. is bodily weak and the 6. was prematurely born.

Among the 50 children of married alcoholics — patients of the Lunatic Asylum in Zurich — STUCHLIK (1915) finds only 28 healthy children (56 %); 5 (10 %) are epileptic, 4 (8 %) are alcoholic or are ailing in some way or other and 13 (26 %) were still-born or died early. PREISIG and AMADIAN (1918) give a list of the illnesses which occurred with 418 descendants (youthful persons and adults) of 100 cured alcoholics.

They refrain from making any comment, as these persons were not personally observed by them. These data under the circumstances cannot be taken into consideration (p. 50).

POLISCH (1927) observed the offspring of sufferers from delirium tremens. Such persons suffered from the effects of chronic alcoholism several years (at least five) before delirium tremens set in. The material concerned is for 74 patients and 58 patients with children. It covers principally alcoholics employed in the alcohol trade without gross psychopathic characteristics. Of 123 children, older than one year five succumbed to infectious diseases in childhood and one died as result of an accident. 70 of the 118 survivors were observed by POLISCH after the fifteenth year. He examined these descendants from delirants for psychoses, epilepsy and psychopathy. POLISCH knew his material personally (page 51). The patients in consequence of previous investigations are not only known phaenotypically but also more or less genotypically.

Of the 70 survivors mentioned most of them were more than 25 years old. One of them was suspected of suffering from epilepsy, having had convulsions in his 2nd year but not later. POLISCH found psychical deficiency among the 123 descendants seven times, but no cases of psychosis and not even one drinker. Only of one person is it reported that he occasionally enjoyed drinking. The descendants were quite fit for society and the state of their health was good.

PANSE (1929) collected material of alcoholics who in their marriage had drunk some time. "Alcoholic", "pre-alcoholic" and "post-alcoholic" children can be distinguished here. PANSE undertook these investigations following the example of BRATZ. In similar material of BRATZ's (communicated by PANSE) comprising 100 fathers, the children were examined for large series of modifications. It was found that alcoholic children are to be distinguished from pre- and post-alcoholic children by smaller length of body and inhibition of the whole body in their youth; also by great morbidity and mortality. The differences are no longer present at the 12th year or at the latest the 14th year.

DITTLER (1922 cit. PANSE) investigated 13 such families and 73 children. He found with "alcoholic" children more debility, inhibition in length, psychopathy and headache, also more epilepsy.

PANSE could only collect 8 similar families with the aid of the

Blue Cross Society. He did not find blastophthory with "alcoholic" children.

PANSE (1929) moreover investigated from this point of view the descendency of 200 serious chronic alcoholics. The ascendents were also examined. There were 780 pregnancies, 12 twins, 71 abortions and 721 normal timely births. Before alcoholism of the father, there were of these 264 children born (and 22 abortions) and during the alcoholism 457 children (and 49 abortions). PANSE found in respect to the occurrence of epilepsy, imbecility and idiocy, psychoses and malformations no difference in number with the praealcoholic and the alcoholic children and concludes the absence of germ injury. Children with modifications (all the said modifications together) PANSE found among the prealcoholic in 10.2 % and among the alcoholic in 10.7 % of the cases. If debility is also included, the figures are successively 19.3 % and 21.8 %. These are high figures. The result is important. If there is indeed a certain distinction between prealcoholic, thus children in the time the father did not drink and alcoholic children i.e. children in the time the father drank then the high percentage refers to the great hereditary transmission of this hospital material and the result is also an indication that similar high percentages which were found by other investigators for all children of alcoholics (thus without distinction of a prealcoholic period) also especially refer to hereditary transmission and less to blastophthory.

The difficulty is however the demarcation line with the father of an alcoholic and a non-alcoholic period. The distinction by PANSE is not prominent; he distinguishes children which were born in a period when alcohol was regularly used in excess and children which were born before that period. PANSE endeavours to establish the beginning of the actual abuse of alcohol. Before that time the fathers however also consumed alcohol. The wives were, except in single cases very moderate in using alcohol.

It is questionable whether this distinction of BRATZ' and PANSE however interesting it may be from a theoretical point of view, is of practical use for the investigation of the action of parental alcoholism.

PANSE (1929) finds in his material a rather great mortality of babies; 19.7 % for prealcoholic children and 16.8 % for alcoholic children (see page 14). There are further a great number of sucklings which died successively from convulsions or suffered from the same.

This refers to a group of children which were born in the years of alcoholism of the father. Also in respect to rachitis PANSE found high figures. He thinks to explain this by the influence of environment. He does not find among children of alcoholic fathers greater morbidity nor greater mortality for tuberculosis (p. 55).

PANSE (1929) in his material refrained from investigating the capability of daughters of alcoholics to feed their children because the will to feed the children is small and it makes investigations impossible (page 56). He does not find in his material a general decline of the social niveau of the children of alcoholic fathers.

Boss (1929) compares the 1016 surviving children of 489 male alcoholics who in their ascendency have no psychopaths and no insanes with children of stigmatized alcoholics, who either themselves are psychopaths or have psychopaths in their ascendency (p. 53) and finds

	debility	psychop.	bodily weak	healthy
Alcoholism only	1.4 %	1.0	1.9	95.7
Stigmatized	7.—	6.2	3.2	83.5

In total Boss finds in the first group 14 debile children and 10 children with other mental defects.

In order to judge of these results it is important to know that of the alcoholics-only, 17 % of the fathers had been able to learn with difficulty at school. It is also ramarkable that inferior children appear together in a few families; e.g. a dem. praecox patient, a schizoide and two debile children occur in one family. The mother is not intelligent and is peculiar.

Summarizing we also find here divergent results. ECHEVERRIA, DEMME, LEGRAIN, SICHEL and STUCHLIK find with children of alcoholics striking mental and physical deviations. We must bear in mind that SICHEL and STUCHLIK observed the descendants of patients of a lunatic asylum who had made an excessive use of alcohol before being taken up. The investigations made by POLISCH are important, yet the result of previous investigations cannot be ruled out by these. POLISCH's material is selective material (see page 51).

Some investigators found very few deviations in the descendants of alcoholics. RÜDIN and WAUSCHKUHN (page 27) ROSENBERG, and SCHWEIGHÖFER met very few cases of epilepsy among children of alcoholics; others found many (p. 32 tab. 3) whilst in the ascendancy of epileptics alcoholism is mentioned very generally. Should there upon further investigations appear to be a difference here, then we should have to take it that alcoholism together with something else in the constitution of patient, would lead to the appearance of epilepsy and other diseases.

The investigations of PANSE are important but it is uncertain, whether the statistical method is of use here. Careful observations retain their value.

14. The Part Heredity, Germ-injury and Effects of Environment have in the Significance of Parental Alcoholism

The investigation of the ascendancy of sufferers from epilepsy, imbecility and idiocy, insanity and nervous diseases, malformations, alcoholism and tuberculosis, teaches us that there is there a frequency of alcoholism. The results of various investigations are very divergent. Of some deviations epilepsy e.g. the connection with alcoholism of the parents is more generally admitted than for others, such as insanity. In this respect we must take into consideration that retrospective information about alcoholics in the ascendancy and information about alcoholism of relatives in general, is difficult to judge as to its value. After the review of the investigations of each of the defects named we have already given our opinion of their significance. We repeat that according to us, with regard to the appearance of the defects, importance must be attached to the connection of the frequent occurrences of alcoholism in the parents with the occurrence of many of the defects named of the children.

Environment, tradition, bad example are significant for the occurrence of alcoholism in the children. This is clear where we encounter a very high percentage of alcoholism in the ascendancy of alcoholics (MINOR, PREISIG and AMADIAN, POLISCH p. 50).

The influence of predisposition and environment are also especially prominent in the Jukes family, the Zero family, the Kallikak family and family number 136. With the Jukes family the influence of environment and tradition is predominant, with the Kallikak family predisposition and heredity.

Environment has also its significance in respect to the occurrence of tuberculosis (p. 55) and perhaps also of epilepsy. (Persons from surroundings where alcohol is used will also use alcohol and the use of alcohol directly induces the occurrence of epilepsy; MUSKENS). Likewise from ROSENBERG's investigations (1913) on the Amberger in the 19th century, the significance of disposition and environment is shown. Of the 18 innkeepers 12 drink heavily, 4 are moderate (2 unknown). That men drink more frequently than women is also generally viewed as an expression of tradition and environment. KROON sees in this a case of sex-limited inheritance (page 47).

ECHEVERRIA has already said (1881 page 502) "that neurotic heredity contributes to a larger extent than vice itself and misery to the widespread of drinking" and LASÈGUE's well known saying „he does not drink who has a will not to drink (ne boit pas qui ne veut) has been repeatedly cited by many French writers. Yet this conclusion which says that an alcoholic is by disposition a psychically degenerate person may not be placed in the foreground too much. The hereditary transmission of alcoholics is generally not found to be higher than 50 %. Environment is also of great importance. We repeat that men drink much more frequently than women and especially in some trades much is drunk. Therefore not every alcoholic is inferior by disposition.

The opinion of PEARSON (page 12) and of PEARL that abuse of alcohol (see later) acts as a selective agent, which has been expressed before their time in the words „l'alcohol elimine la canaille" (alcohol eliminates rabble) is refuted by PREISIG. He says that the effect of alcohol is more like a spreading infection than a selective agent. Alcoholism does not disappear of its own accord.

That some persons show no deleterious physical or mental effects from alcoholabuse is a phaenomenon that in respect to poisons is generally observed (see later, EHRLICH „poison proof").

It is difficult to differentiate between the part of germ poisoning and of pure heredity in parental alcoholism. Various investigators (see the tables and LUNDBORG table 8) mentioned the cases in their statistics where alcoholism was present in the ascendancy only. In those cases it is probable, but not necessary that we are involved in

cases of germ injuries through alcohol. WAGNER-JAUREGG (1928) sees
the effect of germ poisoning in the fact, that alcoholism and
syphilis of the parents have a great part in the ascendance of
patients from dementia praecox according to the investigations
of RÜDIN and of PILCZ. LENZ (1922) accepts an idiokinetic (geno-
typic) effect of alcohol and beside this parakinetic (phaenotypic)
effects, which latter might be expected especially from the mother's
side.

The effects of germ injuries have to be considered differently from
those of pure heredity. For so far as the occurrence of alcoholism in
the ascendancy of alcoholics rests with heredity, we have simply to
do with a hereditary inclination for alcoholic beverages; with alcoholism through blastophthory of the parents the individual is inferior, which is expressed here by lesser will power against alcoholic
temptation and by other defects. Germ injury can create also, I think,
a general inferiority of the brains, through which epilepsy and other
illnesses (p. 42) are facilitated.

Scandinavian investigators GADELIUS (1907 a.o.) point out the
high percentage of insane persons in Sweden i.e. 7 $^o/_{oo}$ and question if
in this we must see the after effects on the germ plasma of the population of the large use of alcohol by the last generation. PROF. LUND-
BORG was so kind as to inform me in reply to my request, that
according to his opinion the statistics covering the number of insane
persons in Sweden do not give a correct idea of the actual ratio. And
the records about this in earlier times are still more uncertain. According to PROF. LUNDBORG it is not possible to say that the percentage of mental defectives was higher formerly (about 1900) than now.
SIOLI (cit. STÜBER) points out that, while the congenital defective
psychoses with Jews appears more frequently than with the rest of
the German population, epilepsy and especially the forms of epilepsy
from birth are fewer (also BRATZ and VOGT, p. 22 and 25). The rarity
of epilepsy with Jews may be explained through the little use of alcohol. There may here however be a question of difference in race.

Concluding we may say that the descendancy of alcoholics may
teach us something more about the significance of parental alcoholism for diseases and inferiority of the children. But especially if we
know also the hereditary characteristics, thus the genotype of the
parents. We must therefore trace also in the ascendancy of the par-

ents the occurrence of diseases (epilepsy, weakmindedness and such like, page 35).

To a certain extent the investigations of DEMME (1890 page 67) comply with this condition and also those of POLISCH (1927c).

It is certainly striking that POLISCH in his material of sufferers from delirium tremens (page 70) finds so few indications of inferiority among the offspring. The material is selective, families with marked symptoms of inferiority have not been included. The investigations would thus especially show the significance of blastophthory. We must however take into consideration the fact that the material also in this sense is selective, that it deals with sufferers from delirium tremens. Sufferers from delirium tremens take a special place among chronic alcoholics. (DRESEL, POLISCH). The results of POLISCH are important; they represent the results of an excellent investigation of scarce material. But besides this we shall also continue to attach value to the many other investigations discussed herein and which indicate the significance of parental alcoholism for the appearance of diseases in children.

Conclusion.

In judging the publications on alcoholism the time of their appearance must be taken into consideration (The truth is the daughter of he time). After the defeat of 1870, there arose in France the necessity of increasing the strength of the nation and idealists then pointed out the danger of parental alcoholism for posterity. TAGUET (1877) begins his publication with a citation from MONTESQUIEU: „La puissance d'une nation dépend du nombre d'hommes valides qu'elle peut appeler sous les drapeaux lorsqu'elle èst menacée". And in general there was a time that medical men were inclined to indicate the abuse of alcohol, also parental abuse of alcohol, as a cause of illnesses. Now the scale has perhaps turned somewhat strongly to the other side and too little value is attached to alcoholism as aetiological moment for diseases (page 111). Our final judgment, as to the significance of parental alcoholism for the children, formed from observations and investigations with human beings, is that there is an injurious effect in different ways and of different degrees of certainty.

The average smaller body weight at birth and in the first few years of development, high infantile death rate, smaller number of healthy adults, indicate a direct injury to the germ plasm through the use of alcohol by the parents. The occurrence of abortion, convulsions, imbecility, malformation, although less definitely known, will also be resultant on this. The occurrence of alcoholism in the ascendancy of sufferers from epilepsy, imbecility and idiocy, insanity and alcoholism and of these diseases in the descendancy of alcoholics points to heredity and germ injury; especially to germ injury if alcoholism in the ascendency is the only hereditary influence and also if the alcoholics, whose descendants show the diseases mentioned, have genotypically no hereditary defects.

One finds some instances described that in families where the parents are drinkers, the children of the successive generations are able to hold their own in society and show no signs of degeneration (alcohol-"proof" EHRLICH).

Clinical observations (i.e. a thorough analysis of single cases) and statistical investigations remain of importance. With statistical investigations, investigations of healthy persons, thus control material, are very necessary. Investigations of families and demographic investigations of small territories must rank foremost (p. 111).

II. Experimental Investigations

By means of experiments with animals investigators have for a long time tried to show the injury to the progeny in consequence of the use of alcohol.

MAIRET and COMBEMALE (1899) gave a dog absinthe during 8 months. In an intermediate period of 8 days it was mated with a dog not treated with alcohol. Twelve young dogs were born, two were still born, seven died of intestinal trouble, epileptic attacks and tuberculosis and three died in consequence of accidents. Another dog was treated with absinthe only during gestation. Of a litter of 6 pups three were still born. Two were normal, but very intelligent and a third was backward in development and growth. This young dog received no alcohol and was mated with a normal dog and bore three pups. One was deformed and died within a few hours, the second died after a fortnight from exhaustion. The third was alive (seven weeks old) and intelligent but had some physical defects.

BOURNÉVILLE and later on BALLET and FAURE, who intoxicated marmots and dogs with alcohol and absinthe found that not one of the progeny remained alive, all died within a few weeks from convulsions (cit. FERRARI 1910). The experiments that were made with dogs by BRATZ and HEBOLD (1901) in order to obtain through chronic alcoholic poisoning progeny with epileptic fits, had negative results. CENI (1905) gave fowls (hens and cocks) 2 years consecutively small quantities of alcohol of 50 % strength. The females laid fewer eggs than the controlled animals (48 : 120), 130 eggs of treated animals brought after 90 to 100 hours incubation 56 (43 %) normal embryos which remained behind in their development. 407 eggs of controlled animals brought 316 (77.6 %) normal embryos. The eggs of treated fowls showed less resistance against the fluctuations of warmth. Ten eggs of treated fowls were normalily incubated. There were 5 infertile eggs, the 5 survivors were weak chickens of which 2 died a few days later, while the other three remained weak creatures. Deformities of all kinds were met with.

BLUHM (1908) finds as expression of constitutional degeneracy of the offspring, a lesser fertility of the young of alcoholized rats. She also finds impotency with drinking male rats.

FERRARI (1910) gave guinea pigs, 2 couples, alcohol per os and to 3 couples subcutan (1.4 cc alcohol per 1 KG body weight, increasing to 2.8 cc.), In the first series one pair was infertile. The second pair produced a litter of 4 young which showed no defects. In the 2nd test the test animals declined very much through the subcutane administration of alcohol. Two pair were infertile. The third pair produced a litter of 4 and 3 young respectively. These offspring showed by microscopic investigations defects in the central nervous system, especially in the spinal cord and corresponding with the defects found in the parents. The mate of this pair showed towards the end of her life epileptic convulsions, likewise one of the young.

KERN (1916) experienced a higher death rate among the offspring of alcoholised guinea pigs than among control animals. Eight surviving young were infected with tuberculosis by KERN, also an equal number of offspring from control mothers. The young of alcoholised mothers succumbed to the infection three days earlier than the control offspring (page 55).

PFÖRRINGER (1912) gave dogs early every day 100—200 ccm.

25—40 % alcohol, according to the size of the animal. He found with the offspring epileptic convulsions, premature births and still births. Fits with dogs of alcoholised parents are also reported by other investigators. (COMBEMALE, HODGE cit. HOPPE).

SCHRÖDER (1913) made experiments during 4 years with rabbits and obtained 6 generations with a total of 100 animals. The rabbits were given alcohol in their food and were drunk at least once per day. Alcohol was adminstered to the young animals from the 4th week of their birth. The alcoholisation is heavy. In order to prevent too great a death rate and in order to obtain sufficient progeny, the administration of alcohol was occasionally stopped. For the rest SCHRÖDER exercised in his tests selection, because he chose the weakest animals for further propagation.

SCHRÖDER finds in this material of rabbits just as among human beings in families where generation upon generation drink, great morbidity, a frequency of backwardness in growth and in the development of the young, high death rate, small offspring, neglect and cases of mothers eating their young. The effect varies very much. Some litters are well developed others are very bad and these also remain defective in their further growth. (1912, p. 734). Of malformations, cataract is mentioned. Convulsions were only observed once.

A disadvantage of these experiments is that no control observations were made, though some writers remark that the treated animals were known with regard to the condition of the young in the time before the experiments were made.

LAITINEN (1908—1926) made experiments with rabbits, guinea pigs and pigeons. LAITINEN gave his test-animals alcohol through the mouth with the help of a stomach tube. The animals get 0.5 ccm³ per kilo animal weight. LAITINEN finds with alcoholised animals a larger total number of young than with control animals. There is a great death rate during the first few days. In a series of experiments with small quantities of alcohol given to guinea pigs there was a death rate of 37% still born and deaths during the first few days, and for control animals a rate of 22 %. In the case of rabbits the death rate was very high, yet the differences were small; 61 % infant mortality for treated animals and 54 % for control animals. With regard to the surviving offspring the average weight of the young of treated rabbits three days after birth was 79 grammes and 88 grams for those of non-treated parents. For guinea pigs the figures are 73 and 77. In the first twenty days, the young of treated rabbits grew at the rate of 7.13 grammes per day, the young of control rabbits 9.46 grammes. For guinea pigs the figures for the first 10 and 20 days are 3.76 gr. and 4.30 gr. for the young of treated parents and 4.12 gr. and 5.20 for the young of control parents. The average increase of weight of the young of treated guinea pigs in the first 110 days was 4.30 gr., for non-treated animals 5.50 gr. These experiments comprise 70 animals, and including the young 348 animals.

At the international Anti-Alcohol Congress of Dorpat in 1926, LAITINEN stated that the experiments with guinea pigs which were continued by him 20 years long, have taught him that alcohol in small quantities 0.2 ccM^3 per kilogramme animal weight has a detrimental effect on the progeny, and which continues for generations (see further page 100).

So far as the said experiments are concerned, alcohol was administered sometimes to the female alone, before or after mating and sometimes to both parents.

FÉRÉ (1893) placed fowls eggs under a dome where alcohol was vaporised. After a day or more the eggs were placed in the incubator. FÉRÉ thus studied the influence of alcohol on the developing germ. He finds that there is a serious retardation of development and the occurrence of monstra. If the eggs are subjected to a long alcohol fumigation, development is stopped altogether.

He considers his findings wholly in conformity with the occurrence of sterility, abortus and malformations among human beings under the influence of alcohol.

In a second experiment, whereby eggs were placed in alcoholic fumes for some time, FÉRÉ (1899) moreover investigated the effects on the later development during a period of rest, which followed the alcoholisation before the stay in the thermostat. Table 9 shows the result. We see that alcoholisation gives a smaller number of normal embryos and indicates a retarded development. The period of rest after alcoholisation appears to increase the injury to the developing embryos. There is a smaller number of normal embryos, yet the degree of development is sometimes higher than with control animals. FÉRÉ sees in this result the expression of the power of variability that under external influences, in one instance may increase, in another instance retard the development, or may produce malformations.

FÉRÉ (1896) turned his experiments in still another direction.

TABLE 9. After FÉRÉ (1899). 72 HOURS INCUBATION

Experiment.	N. of eggs.	Controls.			Alcoholatmosphere.				Alcoholatmosphere and repos.				
		norm embr.	%	state of development	Time of alcoholiz.	norm. embr.	%	state of development	Time of alcoholization	repos	norm. embr.	%	state of development
1	24	20	83.3	48h.15m.	24 h.	19	79.2	42h.15m.	24 h.	24 h.	14	58.3	47h.45m.
2	21	17	81	49h.45m.	48 h.	12	57.1	42h.	48 h.	48 h.	9	42.9	51h.15m.
3	21	18	85.7	44h.	72 h.	13	61.9	37h.30m.	72 h.	72 h.	5	23.8	36h.30m.
4	24	19	79.2	49h.45m.	96 h.	9	37.5	26h.	96 h.	72 h.	1	4.2	52h.
5	24	19	79.2	47h.15m.	96 h.	9	37.5	40h.30m.	96 h.	96 h.	4	16.7	38h.30m.

By making a small opening in the eggshell without reaching the air chamber, he injected several liquids into the egg just as Et. Geoffroy St. Hilaire did long before him according to his son Is. Geoffroy St. Hilaire (1836, III, 501). When he injected aethyl-alcohol he found with 84 treated eggs, 55 normal embryos, i.e. 65.5 %. With 72 control eggs (injected with water) he found 58 normal embryos i.e. 80.6 %.

Two chickens which survived 54 and 57 days, were smaller than the normal (1894). Of all the treated chickens FÉRÉ has only been able to rear one to an adult. (1895, p. 537).

MIRTO gave injections to fowls eggs in the same manner as FÉRÉ and brooded them in the natural way. Of the 18 eggs there were 10 normal chickens, the same number as with eggs injected with water (thus control material). FÉRÉ (1900) compares his results with those of MIRTO and ascribes the great number of non-normal developments which MIRTO obtained by injecting with indifferent substances, to natural breeding. The hen did not treat the injected eggs as intact eggs. STOCKARD (1912) repeated FÉRÉ's experiments and could confirm his results.

STOCKARD (1910) placed eggs of the marine fish Fundulus heteroclitus, a minnow, in solutions of alcohol of different strength (3—9 %). There appeared to be a great individual variability in the manner in which the eggs reacted to the solution. There are many deformations in the development. The alcohol concentration is higher than that which the human being can stand in the blood (page 3).

LAITINEN (1926) finds that the development of frogs eggs in a solution of 0.05 % alcohol is clearly retarded (this seems a very weak solution).

In an other series of experiments made by other investigators the action of alcohol on the spermatozoids has been studied.

KÖLLIKER (1856) already found that alcohol acts detrimentally on the spermatozoids of the bull.

GÜNTHER (1907) investigated besides several other chemical substances, also the action of alcohol on sperma. He made only one test with aethylalcohol with the sperma of a dog which had become weak by standing two hours. He found that motility subsided in 1 % aethylalcohol after 80 minutes. The action of aethylalcohol in the test is weaker than that of other alcohols.

O. HERTWIG (1912) found in his investigations about the changes of the spermatozoids of Rana fusca through chemical substances, which appeared from the disturbances in the development of the normal eggs fertilized by him, that a stay of 2 or 3 hours in 5 % aethyl or methylalcohol does not interfere with later development (page 103). The motility of the spermatozoids under the microscope is just as good if not better than the control material in physiological salt solution.

IVANOW (1913) placed spermatozoids of mammals in an alcohol solution (to 7 %) and investigated the fertilisation afterwards. He found that a stay of half an hour in a weak alcohol solution brought about no injury to the spermatozoids of rabbits and guinea pigs (see further page 103).

It has been thought that the experiment might be able to especially show in how far alcohol directly injures the germs. American investigators have made these experiments especially to obtain in this manner hereditary changes.

In our introduction (page 3) we stated that alcohol, as man uses it, goes for the greater part into the blood. All organs, therefore the sexual glands as well, i.e. the germ gland cells, further the sex cells, the fertilised germ and the foetus in utero are reached and influenced by the alcohol which is in the blood.

NICE (1912, 13, 17) undertook three series of experiments with white mice. In two of these experiments he gave a small quantity of alcohol, 2 ccM^3 of 35 % daily in the food, a quantity whereby the animals remained healthy. This manner of administering alcohol is rather uncertain.

The third time NICE followed the alcohol inhalation method (page 85). The experiments refer to small numbers and the animals are not examined beforehand as to size and frequency of litters and to body weight of the adults and the young. In these experiments therefore the total effect of alcohol on the germ cells and the embryo is studied .In his first experiments the alcoholised animals became heavier than the control animals. In a second experiment, where NICE studied the activity of alcoholised animals, the treated animals had finally a smaller body weight than the control animals. In the alcohol inhalation experiments the alcoholised adults increased less in weight than the control animals. Two of the 4 animals died in the second experiment. Alcohol appears to have had a marked injurious effect on the viability and activity of the mice.

NICE finds that the death rate among the young of alcoholised parents is greater than among that of control animals and that the fertility is also greater. It is important to note that there was not one single death among the control animals (cf. later). The alcoholised animals have larger litters and the number of litters is also greater (not in the second generation). After deducting the number of deaths, the number of mice of treated animals is still larger than with the control mice; there is therefore a larger birth surplus. It is strange to hear that the control mice had few young and many were eaten.

In his first experiments the mean weight of the young of treated parents is greater than of non-treated parents. These young grew quickest when they themselves did not get alcohol. Control animals grew slowest. No young of the alcohol line were deformed, none were born dead and no abortus occurred. In the 3rd experiment with alcohol inhalation, the growth of the young was rather irregular. When they are 8 weeks old, the mean weight of the control young is lower than that of the young of alcoholised parents; at birth it was somewhat higher. According to my opinion not much importance is to be attached to the difference of growth in NICE's experiments. The numbers are small and the results with individuals of a similar line differ considerably.

NICE finds, as LAITINEN (page 79) an increased fertility and a greater infantile mortality. If we can conclude from NICE's experiments that the young in the alcohol line grow well, then this result, cannot be attributed to selection, according to PEARL (page 87). In this manner the weak germs would have died through alcoholisation. There were no abortions and stillborn. NICE mentions only the young, which died from lack of viability; he however does not state how long after birth death took place. Not one of the control young succumbed. In cases where the number of births and also the birth surplus is larger in the alcohol line than in the control line, one can hardly define the fact that in the alcohol line there are deaths and in the control line there are no deaths of young, whilst the body weight of the young in the alcohol line is greater than in the control line (how great the weight is of the young of the alcohol line which die is not mentioned) as being a selective action of alcohol. (PEARL 1924 p. 20). At birth, thus before death of the young the average weight of the alcohol line was already greater than that of the control line. This was not the case in the 2nd generation which had also been subjected to alcohol. Of these young the body weight increased in 8 weeks to more than that of the control young. The signification of NICE's experiments is very restricted in connection with the alcohol. It is to be mentioned that in the control line of both experiments (1912, 17) not one of the animals died, whilst in the alcohol line the death rate was 11.1 % (9 : 81), in the first generation and 12.5 % (7 : 56) in the second generation and in the experiment of 1917, 6 %, 9.8 % and 6 %. (Cf. also the critic of STOCKARD, 1912).

The results of the experiments of different investigators are not in conformity. Different dosage is also of importance. AGNES BLUHM (1921) alcoholised white mice by giving them every other day 0.2 ccM³ of a 20 % alcohol solution, by means of an injection under the skin of the back. In this experiment the alcohol intoxication was very severe. Also in this proof the total parental alcoholism is studied (p.82). The number of sterile matings is great. There is a smaller number of litters with treated animals than with control animals, also the litter is smaller. If the females have been alcoholised, the differences are much greater than when the male is alcoholised. The young are often dead and badly developed. In an exceptional case, i.e. in one litter of two young, these individuals are strong and have resisting power.

COLE and DAVIS (1914) made the following experiments with rabbits. When two bucks are mated with one doe superfoetation is frequent and one can see that one of the bucks is father of most of the young of one litter. Such a buck with prominent propagatory power was exposed to alcoholic inhalation for a month or so. There was then not one young of his in the next litter. As only mated he shows fertility. We see here therefore also a weakening effect of the physiological behaviour of the spermatozoids through a short alcohol treatment, which is to be compared with the reduced number of fructations with stronger alcohololisation of the experiments with Rana by BILSKI (page 103). From this experiment appears the injurious effect of the alcohol on the male sexual organs.

STOCKARD (1912) administered alcohol first by making his test animals, guinea pigs, inhale alcohol. Through the inhalation method the animals are placed in an alcohol atmosphere; during the first few years of the experiment one hour daily, later years, the males two hours and the females three hours, six days of the week. The animals may remain until they are completely intoxicated or they may be only affected to such an extent that they still attempt to walk. The amount of treatment employed however, does not produce complete intoxication. Characteristic of this method is that narcosis only lasts a short time in contrast with drunkenness, which is the consequence of imbibing through the mouth. The animals remained absolutely healthy and lived long (page 9). The use of alcohol according to the inhalation method cannot simply be compared with the use of alcohol through the mouth. In the latter case there is a chronic damage to the tissues of the digestive tube with injurious effect on the organism (see also STOCKARD 1918 page 139). The object of STOCKARD's experiments was to study the action of alcohol on the male sex cells and on the female sex cells and the developing fruit, separately (page 82).

STOCKARD carried on his experiments for thirteen years and the records cover 5000 animals (1924). It represents the greatest test material which the alcohol literature contains. From the different tables of STOCKARD's publications it appears that with alcoholised animals the average litter is smaller than with control animals. The small size of litter is reached owing to the fact that with alcoholised animals among the litters which comprise 1—5 young, more small

litters occur and this is partly due to death of embryos. These prenatal deaths have been carefully studied by STOCKARD.

The large number of small litters with alcoholised animals is due to
so many prenatal deaths in the large litters and partly to reduced
sexual activity, thus to reduced fructation. The number of matings
not followed by gravidity is greater with alcoholised animals than
with control animals. The number of young which became adults is
smaller for alcoholised parents than for control parents. One must
here compare the totals for the same size of litters. When alcoholised animals produce large litters the animals are in an exceptionally
bad condition. The mortality is larger with the young of alcoholised
parents than of control animals. We must in this respect not lose
sight of the fact that the number of small litters with alcoholised
parents is larger than with control parents. This circumstance makes the total infantile mortality with alcoholised parents smaller.

Infantile mortality is calculated by STOCKARD from the whole alcoholised stock. If one calculates it from the F_1 generation thus for
the young from alcoholised parents the ratio is 189 : 100. Further
the prenatal mortality is largest and the infantile mortality takes
place during the first few days after birth. Among the young of alcoholised animals $2\frac{1}{2}$ % monstrous animals with great defects are
met with. No monsters occur among the young of control animals.
That the general physical condition of the young of control animals is
better than that of alcoholised animals, also appears from the fact
that animals with a large body weight at the age of three months
(when becoming adults) appear in $5\frac{1}{2}$% of the total among the young
from control parents and in $2\frac{1}{2}$ % of those of alcoholic parents.
Among the latter there are more with an excess weight.

The average weight of the new born of control animals and of alcoholised parents, for each litter is 197 and 165 grammes respectively
and per offspring 7 and 70 grammes. When the young are a month
old the figures are 228.6 grammes and 214 grammes and when they
are three months old 425 and 404 grammes. The differences, says
STOCKARD, are smaller in later years than they were in the first
years, especially as a result of better treatment which was greatly
beneficial to the weak animals of alcoholised parents.

Illustrative for STOCKARD's results is also table 10, which refers to
matings in the years 1919/21 with non-treated animals which were

TABLE 10. ALTERNATE MATINGS OF NORMAL ANIMALS WITH NORMAL AND ALCOHOLIC MATES. (Tab. 1. STOCKARD, 1922 and 1924, experiment 1919—1921)

	Matings of 35 Normal Males, successively with		Matings of 44 Normal Females, successively with	
	Normal Females	Treated Females	Normal Males	Treated Males
Number of matings .	81	81	77	81
Total offspring . . .	196 2,42 Av.lit.	185 2,28 Av.lit.	195 2,53 Av.lit.	182 2,25 Av.lit.
Failure to conceive .	6 7,90 %	6 7,90 %	3 3,89 %	10 12,34 %
Lived over 3 months	151 77,03 %	105 56,64 %	161 82,56 %	118 64,83 %
Died under 3 months	45 22,96 %	80 43,35 %	34 17,45 %	64 35,16 %
Defective	0	11 5,95 %	0	9 4,97 %

alternately mated with non-treated and treated animals. A similar table has been published in 1918 of the 6th and 7th year of the experiments.

PEARL (1916/1917) takes fowls for his experiments following the methods of STOCKARD by subjecting them to aethylalcohol, methylalcohol or aether fumes. At the outset he has two breeds some specimen of which were alcoholised, he investigated the F_1 animals and speaks of possibilities about F_2 animals.

PEARL's great plan has only been carried through to a small extent. He set forth the results for more than a year in a series of three publications. Later on he published a part of the results for the year following and then the experiments stopped. (PEARL 1924).

PEARL says that these results clearly indicate germinal selective action. Selective action is a strong argument for evolution; it is however often only accepted and not proved. Selective action may be concluded from PEARL's experiments, but the question is whether these experiments admit such conclusions (Cf. page 145). Indeed there are many imperfections to be found in these experiments. Care should be taken as to the correct dosage. The three animals treated with methylalcohol died because they were treated too long in the cage. Four animals treated with aether died for the same reason. In 1915 there was exceptionally great mortality among chicks owing to some infectious diseases. When mating it appeared that the control cock was sterile. In these experiments therefore there were no matings of a non-treated cock with a treated hen and also there were no control matings. There were apparently no prelimanary experiments undertaken to establish fertility. The treated animals were weighed weekly but the control animals only occasionally. The care of the chicks was left to a new servant who did not look after them properly. Not all chicks after hatching were kept. The totals are often small and the matings of the same groups show very divergent results. Percentages of very small numbers are calculated; very divergent totals are included and average figures are found without it having been taken into consideration whether this would be permitted statistically [1]).

The significance of the results therefore must be accepted with reserve. If the experiments had been prolonged for a longer period the different failures would have been avoided.

PEARL's results are the following. When mating an alcoholized cock with a non-treated hen, the number of the infertile eggs is just as large as with the control material. There is also nothing to be deduced from the number of chickens which come out as to differences in respect to control animals. (Table 11, p. 90).

It is probable when matings are effected where both parents have been subjected to alcoholic inhalation that the number of infertile eggs is greater than with matings of non-treated animals. Considering

---

[1]) In the group ethyl treated male with untreated female e.g. the number of infertile eggs in three groups is 2,0 and 4, of 20,25 and 33 eggs respectively, of a fourth group it is 17 of 33 eggs. The total deaths in shell is also divergent, three times in agreement 7, 4 and 4 and once divergent namely 22.

In the experiment treated male with treated female the number of infertile eggs in three groups is 15, 20 and 19, of 28, 25 and 27 eggs respectively and in a fourth group divergent namely 2 of 24 eggs.

now the number of eggs which are not hatched (i.e. the foetus that died in the shell) it might be expected that this number would also be much larger. This would have been the case if the injurious action of alcohol had also reached the fertilized germs. This does not appear to have been the case; the number of foetus which die in the shell is small.

As to the death of the chickens it may possibly be deduced for matings of treated and non-treated animals that the death rate does not differ from the normal control material. The death rate of chickens from alcoholised parents is small. It concerns only small figures.

The weight of the chickens at birth shows the same as already found for the number of animals which die in the shell and for the death of the chickens. The average weight of chickens, of which only the father was subjected to alcoholic inhalation, does not differ from the average weight of chickens from non-treated parents which have been brought forward as control material. The average weight of chickens at birth from parents both treated, is higher.

The continued checking of the body weight of the chickens teaches us that the chickens of parents of which one or both were treated with alcohol had a higher average weight than chickens of control material.

Deformations were not more frequent among chickens from alcoholised parents than among normal parents.

The brief communication about the results of 1916 does not justify any change of our opinion of the proving-power of the experiments. The results are divergent. When alcoholising both parents, 18 eggs of 82 were fertile, thus 22 %; when the mother only was alcoholised there were 5 fertile eggs of 63 eggs, i.e. 8 %. In the first case there was a prenatal mortality, (death in shell) of 11 %, in the second case of 80 %. In how far non-alcoholic ancestry is actually control material and not comparison material, such as in 1915, is not reported.

In 1916 the occurrence of malformations was carefully pursued. It appears that there is no difference in respect to the progeny from untreated parents.

From Table 11 it appears that in chickens from matings of which only the cock was alcoholised there are no differences to be seen in

TABLE 11. SHOWING A SUMMARY FROM THE EFFECT OF CONTINUED
ADMINISTRATION OF ALCOHOL BY THE INHALATION METHOD UPON
THE PROGENY. (PEARL'S RESULTS).

Character studied	treated males and untreated femals %	treated males and treated femals %	untreated „controls" ¹) %	Net result on offspring of treated males and untreated females	Net result on offspring of treated males and treated females
1. Percentage of infertile eggs . . .	20.9	53.9	23.3	0	—
2. „ „ embryo dying in shell	42	27.1	42.2	0	+
3. „ „ fertile eggs which hatched	58	72.9	57.8	0	+
4. „ „ all eggs which hatched	45.9	33.7	44.4	0	—
5. „ mortality under 180 days of age	33.3	10.0	36.9	0	+
6. Mortality over 180 days of age .	0 : 28	0 : 27	1 : 41	?	?
8. Mean hatching weight, males . .	34.9 g.	37 g.	34.2 g.	0	+
9. „ „ „ females . .	35.0 g.	27 g.	34.7 g.	0	+
10. „ adult weight, males . . .	2669 g.	2815 g.	2392 g.	+?	+?
11. „ „ „ females . .	2020 g.	2063 g.	1928 g.	+?	+?

respect to comparison material. If both parents are alcoholised, the
number of infertile eggs is very much larger and over against this the
number of chickens which died in the shell is small. The death rate of
the chickens which are hatched is also smaller and the weight of body
is larger.

PEARL. says that alcohol acts as a selective agent on the germ cells
and prevents the formation of offspring, except the strongest and the
most resistent germ cells, and it does not appear that any germ injurious effect has taken place on the sexual cells, which formed
fructified germs.

---

¹) I put controls between brackets, because we have not to do with
control animals strictly speaking (Cf. texte).

²) These data are established from the material of 1913.

PEARL's publications have made a great impression. This was caused by the explanation PEARL gave of his results (p. 87). His explanation agrees with that of PEARSON's. We abide by that which we can deduce from the experiments. The divergent and often small numbers in PEARL's experiments, as stated before, deter us from any far reaching generalisation (see also page 145).

We shall continue the discussions about STOCKARD's experiments. He first gave a description of his experiments in 1912 and 1913, further detailed publications in 1916 and in 1918 and still further information in 1922. It must be said here that the publication of 1918 does not quite correspond with that of 1916.

STOCKARD began his experiments in 1910; the publication for 1916 covers 5 years; the number of animals examined is 700 in four generations. As to the conditions of health of the surviving animals STOCKARD in 1913 said that they were usually small, timid and excitable. The experiments for 1913 cover 42 matings and 9 control matings. There were many cases of abortus and 14 still born. Of the 32 living young, only seven remained; six of these survived, five of which were small for their age and very timid and also excitable. There were many cases of death from convulsions among the young. STOCKARD speaking of the survivors, in his publication of 1916 says that if the sire is alcoholised, nearly all the progeny consist of nervous and excitable animals.

During the first five years of the experiments STOCKARD mated later generations several times, i.e. the young of alcoholised animals (F_1) with each other, or again with other alcoholised animals and also with normal animals. In the next generation (F_2) again the young of alcoholised grandparents were mated together and in other ways. These different matings are mentioned separately. In the succeeding generations there are again many nervous excitable animals (more than half), and deformations are more frequent among the offspring of F_1 and F_2 parents than among the offspring of direct alcoholised animals. The 13 survivors of the third generation were rather weak and degenerate and practically quite sterile. The alcoholised generation appears in this stadium of the experiment to become almost extinct in the fourth generation.

From these observations it is shown that in the experiments during the years 1910—1915 the physical and mental condition of the sur-

vivors was very unfavourable and according to the opinion of
STOCKARD there was an increasing tendency to inferiority.

In the publications of 1918 in respect to this train of thought there
is no continuity. The publication deals with the results of the 6th and
7th year of the experiments. The experiments comprise 1170 guinea
pigs. Breeding was carried on with the same test animals as in the
experiments of 1910—1915, and furthermore in 1915 further new
material was employed. In the years 1916—1917 there were no matings where both parents were alcoholised. Of matings in later generations, matings with the offspring of alcoholised parents and of
grandparents are not mentioned separately. There is a small group
where the male offspring of alcoholised fathers were in their turn alcoholised and mated with normal and further a group where the
female offspring of treated mothers were alcoholised and mated with
normal sires.

During these years there were especially many matings of alcoholised offspring with normal animals. The daily alcoholisation of
alcoholised animals was longer.

STOCKARD in his publications for 1918 accepts the opinion of
PEARL. He writes: "we have a stronger individual selection during the
uterine life so, that the surviving individuals in a given stadium are of
a better average quality than during any previous stadium. The ratio
of the strongest to the weakest animals by reason of this selection
continually tends to increase." It must be considered that this improvement is relative, namely in respect to the very bad beings which
died in the uterus. The question is whether the surviving young of the
alcohol animals are better than those of the control animals. From
the description of the experiments 1910/1915 it is very clear that the
condition of the survivors is bad. The description of the experiments
of 1916/1917 contains indications that the condition of the offspring
is not so good as that of control animals e.g. firstly their weight is
smaller, secondly in large litters of alcoholised parents the offspring
are small and weak, only a few survive and these few survivors remain far behind normal animals from large litters, thirdly in the succeeding generations many deformations are met with, the weight of
the newly born animals is smaller, the prenatal mortality is higher
than normally. Beside this we also come across the simple observation in the publication of 1918 that survivors are capable of a nor-

mal existence. The difference between the results of 1910/1915 and 1916/1917 is especially that the condition of the offspring in later generations in the experiments of 1916/1917 gradually becomes better. STOCKARD ascribes this to better treatment and to mating with normal animals. Especially in the latter way the improvement will be obtained, for as a result of better hygienic measures weaker animals will remain alive and by this the value of the animals would just become less through "contra selection". There would therefore be many nervous and excitable animals. We should like to know how many matings of alcoholized animals were done. There were 28 alcoholized males and 34 alchoolized females in the experiments of the 6th and the 7th year and there are records of 1170 animals.

The brief communications of 1922 and of 1924 do not remove the contrast in the results and in line of thought of the experiments of 1910/1915 and 1916, 1917. STOCKARD mentions in this publication some results of the experiments in the years 1919/1921 covering 1700 animals (according to table 2, 1922). During all the years (1909/1921) of the experiments more than 5000 animals were examined (1924). Particulars of the experiments of 1917 are not mentioned. The treatment of both parents does not greatly alter the results, which have followed if the mother alone had been treated. In this publication STOCKARD simply adheres to the standpoint that alcohol acts as a selective agent, in the sucessive generations in the alcohol line only the best are suitable for producing the following generation, only the most vigorous animals remain for propagation. Considering the successive generations it is seen that the offspring from directly treated parents present the poorest records of all. According to my opinion this may not at all be generalised from the results of the experiments of STOCKARD in 1910/1918. Also in the experiments of 1919/1921 the weight of the newly born animals of the following generations is smaller and the prenatal mortality is larger than normally. From his table No. 2 (1922) it appears that if no alcohol is given in the succeeding generations and if many matings with non-treated animals take place, the average weight of the young gradually increases. In the 5th generation of this experiment (F_4) which comprise a small number of animals (59), the average weight of the offspring is somewhat smaller than the control animals. The size of the litter is smaller the percentage for survivors is somewhat higher. Nothing more is

said of the malformations, which play an important role in STOCK-
ARD's experiments. According to table 10 page 87 (STOCKARD's
table 1, 1922) malformations also occurred in the experiments of
1919/1921. When analysing the successive generations it would be
desirable to have parallel controlmaterial in the manner of MAC
DOWELL's (page 97).

How the gradual improvement in STOCKARD's experiments comes
about further investigation must show. Selection is a plausible explanation. There is selection when the offspring of alcoholized
parents show a higher resistance against alcohol than the original
material. The result of STOCKARD's experiments is more probably
a question of regeneration of the germ cells than of selection. The
result would then signify that the germ plasm is not permanently
injured by the effects of alcohol. This is something which may also be
concluded from the experience of the use of alcohol by man. It has
been said that if it were otherwise, the human race in the case of
general use of alcohol would be harmed still more than is already the
case. Blastophthory is probably a phaenotypical phenomenon (false
heredity of JOHANNSEN).

It is necessary that STOCKARD's experiments be continued and
strictly concentrated upon the investigations of the effects of alcohol.

One would wish that many experiments were made with many
animals of matings of treated male and non-treated female, of non-
treated male and treated female and of treated male and treated
female and also with the same animals, which have been alcoholized
for half a year, a year and longer. One would also wish to see the
alcoholization continued with the offspring of treated animals.

There are still some few experiments to report, in the first place
about experiments with fowls.

PEARL made still another series of experiments (1916b) by ex-
posing eggs in an incubator to alcoholic fumes. Three groups of eggs
were exposed to the alcohol atmosphere, 1, 2 and 3 weeks respectively.
The number of prenatal deaths was slightly higher in the first two
groups and much higher in the third group than with control material.
The number of chickens that came out of the eggs was smallest in the
group most heavily alcoholised. Furthermore a larger number of this
group died than of the other groups with lower dosage and than
those of control animals. There was no question of selection here.

We have already seen that FÉRÉ made similar experiments and reported his results (page 80). There is still a short report of experiments with chickens by VAN DER HOEVEN (1919). His attention is wholly directed towards the influence of alcohol as a racial poison. VAN DER HOEVEN traced not only in how far the germ developed in the egg and whether the living chickens showed numerous deformities, but also how the survivors grew up, how their progeny developed and also how this became with or without renewed alcohol treatment.

VAN DER HOEVEN gives chickens alcohol through the stomach tube and finds that whilst with control experiments only in 12 % of the eggs no development takes place and in also 12% chickens succumb before birth, these figures after the administration of alcohol, rise to 37% and 54%. Whether either the mother or the father or both are alcoholised it makes very little difference. Of 351 alcoholised eggs, only 32 chickens are born alive instead of 266. They are very small, weak in the legs, sickly and badly developed. Several die before they are a few months old. Only a few deformities occur. The bad effect of alcohol is clearly seen in the second and still more clearly in the third generation. Abstinence from alcohol brings about an unexpected speedy improvement.

Here it will be seen that VAN DER HOEVEN's results are not identical with PEARL's (p. 75). VAN DER HOEVEN found a great number of infertile eggs and many cases of death in shell. Furthermore the chickens born were small, weak and sickly.

There is scanty information about VAN DER HOEVEN's experiments. We do not know any details. The observation that it makes very little difference whether the mother or the father or both parents are alcoholised is surprising. The following remark, that Prof. VAN DER HOEVEN wrote to me, is important. When the eggs were brooded to the end, far fewer malformations and failures were found than ST. HILAIRE believed to see, when he opened the eggs after having had the eggs brooded only some days.

HOUWINK (1917) gives the following brief account of experiments in consequence of PEARL's publication of 1916. Each of two groups of one cock and 6 hens, brothers and sisters, laid the first year 160 eggs per hen, which gave 80—85% sound chickens. The second year an increasing quantity of alcohol in the food, 1—30 ccm brandy, was given to one of the two groups during a month; the animals were in the last week quite drunk; the second group served as control animals. These control animals produced the same number of eggs and of chickens as the first year. In the alcohol group sound chickens hatched from eggs of the first week of alcoholisation, in a somewhat higher percentage than the control group (the numbers are not mentioned). The percentage of the fertilization in the 2nd, 3rd and 4th week were respectively 50%, 20% and 0%. Nothing is said of the progress of development and of the state of the chickens hatched. The group that had been alcoholized for a month gave at the beginning of the next laying period eggs that were fertilized in the ordinary way and hatched sound chickens.

This experiments teaches us nothing more than that with increasing alcoholisation of both parents the number of fertilized eggs drops at the end to zero.

Experiments with fowls were also made by DANFORTH (1919), the object being to define wholly the selective effects of certain characteristics and not the deleterious effect on the germ cells. DANFORTH allowed a very long inhalation treatment, viz. of 2 hours, with alternating periods of daily alcohol treatment viz. of 2 hours, with alternating periods of daily alcohol treatment and non-alcohol days as controlling periods. He had the same experience as PEARL, that the duration of treatment becomes rapidly disastrous with fowls. Cocks withstand the treatment better then hens. Of five hens four died in the long run in consequence of treatment.

DANFORTH found a slight decrease of body weight. The data given in the experiments about fertility are rather indefinite and in connection with the purpose of the experiment, probably cannot be compared with PEARL's. DANFORTH did not find in the alcohol period of the experimental animals more infertile eggs than in the control period. There was a large and varying number of offspring which died in the shell and there are no marked differences in the alcohol and control periods.

In the third experiment where the daily inhalation was longest, the number of infertile eggs is larger than in the other experiments. Also in the control period the number of the infertile eggs is great (possibly after effects). The number of young which died in the shell is in this experiment also very great.

This is contrary to the results of PEARL's experiments where both parents were alcoholised and corresponds with those of VAN DER HOEVEN's and CENI's (p. 98).

KOSTITSCH (1922) gave white rats 1.4 ccm alcohol p. die during a long time. The sperm-forming cells of the testicles degenerated, whereas the interstitial ceels were spared. He found disturbances in the nucleus divisions. In the end sterility occurred.

Mac DOWELL's experiments with the inhalation method with albino rats are very important. The experiments were very extensive and very much attention was paid to comparing alcohol material with control material. MACDOWELL tells us that he experienced how small material of unknown origin and nature may lead to an investigator incorrectly ascribing the results to the influence of alcohol, which have nothing to do with the experiment and which depend on the heredity of the material. Therefore good control material is necessary.

MACDOWELL and VICARI studied the intelligence of his experimental animals, that of the "grand-children" of alcoholised rats and found that the posterity of alcoholised grandparents did not withstand intelligence tests (running in a labyrinth) so well as control animals (p.101).

Further, MACDOWELL investigated the fertility and growth of albino rats whilst under the influence of alcohol fumes. He had at his disposal 177 rat couples and 1755 young. The real brothers and sisters and their direct offspring served as control material. There are matings with rats which were treated and whose parents were also treated and of rats which were not treated but whose parents or grand parents were treated.

Compared with control material it appears that in the alcohol material the number of litters and the sizes of the litters are somewhat smaller. The difference occurs in all four groups named.

He found the number of litters per pair of alcoholised animals smaller, particularly small with animals highly alcoholised. The first litter appears later with alcohol animals than with control animals.

Also AGNES BLUHM found a greatly reduced number of matings (page 84) and STOCKARD found a considerable number of unsuccessful matings (page 86).

In the case of treated rats of treated parents MAC DOWELL finds the number of litters somewhat smaller than with control material.

With two other experiment groups, namely with non-treated rats of treated parents and treated grandparents, the number of litters per pair is larger than with control material.

MacDowell attributes this to selection. I should think that only the injurious effect of direct treatment has been demonstrated. The result of the test groups of non-treated rats of treated parents and grandparents is uncertain because the control groups of both these test groups produced different results.

Mac. Dowell rightly points out the great significance of comparable control material. The demand for this has been rigidly adhered to by him. It now appears that material of various experiment groups shows greatly varying results, perhaps by reason of different degrees of inbreeding. The mean number of litters per couple of non-treated rats of treated parents and of non-treated rats of treated grand parents is exactly as large as for control material of the first of these two experimental groups. In view of this it is not necessary to assume any special selection.

Finally, Mac Dowell investigated the growth. The average weight of treated animals weighed at different times is smaller than with control material.Of non-treated animals of treated parents and of treated grandparents these figures are somewhat irregular, yet probably the weight is higher than that of control material. Of treated animals of treated parents the differences are very undecided and slight.

In order to know the significance of alcohol treatment of the parents for the offspring, the weight at birth and during the first few weeks after must in the first place be known. Mac Dowell's data only begin when the animals are 40 days old.

Mac Dowell (1926) and his collaborators defined the prenatal mortality with white mice by determining the difference between the number of corpora lutea of the mother and the size of the litter.

Slight alcoholisation of female mice does not change the prenatal mortality and generally speaking brings about no changes in pregnancy. Heavy alcoholisation increases the prenatal mortality of the embryos. Heavy alcoholisation of the father showed no marked results as to the prenatal death of their litters. One male had no influence whatsoever, whereas another male with the same dame had. Furthermore they found (1926, 1928) that the differences in the prenatal mortality is independent of the difference in sex-ratio at birth. Alcohol treatment has no influence on the sex-ratio of the mouse.

This was found to be otherwise by DANFORTH (page 96) and BLUHM. BLUHM found an increase of the number of males and thinks that the negative result of MAC DOWELL is to be explained by reason of the strong stock used by him, so that the alcohol is quickly secreted and the animals at the time of mating were no longer under the influence of alcohol. This problem has therefore not yet been solved. MAC DOWELL worked with the largest number.

The fact considered here is that where the male mouse has two kinds of sexual cells (for both sexes), perhaps one kind is more susceptable to the influence of alcohol than the other. This will be proved by the changing of the sex ratio. BLUHM found in her first experiment (1923) an important increase of the number of males, in a second exp eriment (1926) this increase was considerably less; she gave them then less alcohol. BLUHM thinks that the paralytic effects of alcohol on the femal determinants of the male sex cells are stronger than on the male determinants. BLUHM 1930, see p. 143 [1]).

HANSON and his collaborators undertook experiments with albino rats using the inhalation method and published various reports in regard to this. (HANSON and HANDY 1923, HANSON and HEYS 1924, 1927, HANSON 1923, 1928). They continued their experiments with inhalation during 10 generations; afterwards they observed the material of several further generations without alcohol treatment. The results are somewhat varying. In their preliminary reports, HANSON and HANDY (1923) mention that in the first generation they found a greatly impaired fertility. Six alcoholic females were mated and in a period of six months only four litters were born. Four of the six animals never produced a litter. Three of these did not show any signs of pregnancy at any time and were rendered completely sterile. The effects of the treatment on the fourth alcoholic female were vastly different. She was pregnant three times and each time the litter was slowly absorbed. She aborted another time. This was followed by three more absorptions. After these matings with an alcoholic male she was mated with a normal male. The following month she gave birth to one still born young. She was then mated with a normal male. The following month she gave birth to one still born young. She was then mated with normal males until her death but showed no further signs of pregnancy. The fifth animal had a litter of five. One died on the first day and the rest died four days later. This animal did not breed again, although she was continually mated up to the time of her death, which took place a year later. The germ cells of one (the 4th female) were so impaired that the only litter she threw died in a few days. The 5th female had suffered less injury, but was not able to bring any of her eight litters, perhaps with the exception of one, to the full term.

The sixth alcoholic female produced all the young that carried on the alcohol line. She threw two litters of normal size and weight and gave birth to one animal, which died on the 3rd day. A fourth litter consisted of six young of normal appearance, thus she produced four litters, of which three were normal. There were 86 control offspring of four productive controls against 26 alcoholics of one alcoholic female. The one fertile alcoholic female therefore proved to be a slightly better breeder than the average of the control animals.

HANSON (1923) found in the 3rd generation all animals to be weak. HANSON and HEYS (1924) found in the first three generations a distinct decrease of the mean weight of body.

In 1927 and 1928 HANSON and HEYS report the results of the experiments during 10 generations, which lasted five years and comprised 1688 treated and 1435 control animals.

There is an average difference of 0.2 grammes between the average weight of the male young of treated and those of control animals. For the successive generations the values are somewhat divergent. At twenty days the young females have a larger mean weight of 0.93 grammes than the control animals.

During treatment the mean weight of the treated animals becomes smaller than for control animals. (HANSON, SHOLES, HEYS, 1928). The litters are larger in the case of treated animals than with control animals.

The average sex ratio is slightly smaller for treated animals than for control animals. (49.4 and 53.1 % males respectively). In 7 of 9 generations (2nd till 10th) this difference is found. After comparing and investigating the differences HANSON and HEYS conclude that there is no alteration of the sex ratio.

Atfer ten years of alcoholic treatment, the descendants that are no longer treated are examined in order to find out the power of resistance against alcohol fumes In the publication of 1927 HANSON and HEYS say that the descendants of the 10th generation were examined by them; in the publication of 1928 they only speak of albino rats which had an alcoholic ancestry of ten generations.

The experience with treated animals was that every animal individually during the course of treatment acquired greater power of resistance; therefore an acquired resistance exists during life.

For their investigations HANSON and HEYS (1927) took 60 rats of the 13th generation (30 descendants, great grandchildren of treated material of the 10th generation and also 30 great grandchildren of control material of the 10th generation).

The result is that the control animals possess greater power of resistance against alcohol fumes than treated animals. The differences are small. The somewhat decreased power of resistance of the young of experiment animals indicates an enfeeblement, therefore germ injury, as BILSKI (page 103) found with frogs.

HANSON and COOPER (1930) have studied In this material whether alcoholism of the ancestors causes psychical changes in the offspring. They investigated the capacity for learning of the animals with the so-called labyrinth. The results are not in conformity and the differences are often small. The authors conclude that there are no real differences; BLUHM (1930) is of the opposite opinion,

The experiment is confusing because HANSON and HEYS' object was to investigate the question of the heredity of acquired characteristics; for this reason they took the great grandchildren of the 10th generation of alcoholics. In view of the effect of alcohol it would have been of special importance to have investigated the children and the grandchildren of the 10th alcohol generation.

A great objection to HANSON and HEYS' experiment is that the whole of the alcohol offspring descends from one alcohol female (see page 99). Of 6 alcoholic females, five dropped off, the sixth proved to be slightly better in breeding than the average control animal.

ROST and WOLF (1925) made some experiments with rabbits. They conducted matings of three treated females and an untreated male, of three untreated females and a treated male and of one treated female and a treated male. In these experiments there were seven alternate periods of alcohol and non-alcohol treatment. Small increasing quantities of alcohol were administered 2—8 ccM^3 pure alcohol per day. In these experiments the writers found no influence on the offspring through parental alcoholism.

Regarding insects, HARRISON (1919) made some experiments with alcohol vapour with the Lepidopterous insect Selenia and MANN (1923) with the banana fly Drosophila.

HARRISON took at the outset 90 fertilised eggs of one couple, using 45 for the alcohol treatment and 45 for control material. Alcohol treatment was severe, the mortality enormous. Seven alcohol Selenia butterflies came out, of which two were defective. The five moths which were obtained from 45 fertilised eggs which were objected to fumesduring the further development were strong animals. They had a larger mean wing span than control animals and furnished very good breeding material which had small mortality, grew rapidly and produced a large new generation of moths.

This fine experiment deals with a small number of animals. HARRISON refers to his publication as being preliminary. The result here may be taken in the same sense as with PEARL and PEARSON, viz that through heavy alcoholisation a great number of germs (in PEARL's case germ cells) succumb during the course of development; only a few fertilised eggs offering very great resistance (5 out of 45) become moths and that these survivors by reason of this resistibility or insusceptibility (alcohol "proof", EHRLICH) are not impaired by the influence of alcohol. They were in several respects the best, viz, in size of body and fertility (p. 145).

MANN (1923) who worked with the Drosophila fly found an increase of broods through alcoholisation of adult animals. There is therefore either an increased sexuality or a favourable influence on the germ cells. The ratio of the insects bred, the number of representants of both sexes, the number of different colours types according to MANN infer that alcoholisation has exercised a favourable influence. The results of MANN's experiments are diametrically opposed to those of HARRISON's as to significance. HARRISON found good animals in his experiments because all weak animals perished. MANN found good animals becauses the germ cells had improved. These investigators followed different methods. HARRISON alcoholised fertilised eggs and during their further development. Mann alcoholised adult animals and studied their posterity. The dosage of alcohol given by HARRISON was very great.

PEARL and ALLEN (1926) placed seeds of the Cucumis Melo for three hours in different solutions of alcohol. The germ percentage is lower than with control material, the growth is better. PEARL sees in the result a selective action.

We must still discuss experiments which were undertaken by BILSKI with frogs and which correspond with those of HERTWIG, STOCKARD, etc. (page 81, 82) already discussed.

BILSKI (1921) placed frogs in a $\frac{1}{2}$—2% solution of alcohol. The blood rapidly takes the same ratio as the surrounding liquid. BILSKI after some time (14 days) collected by operative means, the sex cells and studied the fertilization and the posterity. His object was to cause injuries to the germ cells (before fertilization). There is also here individual variability of tolerance. The modification in development which brings about poisoning of the male are not so great as with the female. Upon slight alcoholisation an increase in the number of embryos is found, the offspring increases and is vigorous. Upon heavy alcoholisation the number of embryos is smaller; sooner or later there is during development an increased falling off of descendants, so that finally the number of survivors is not larger than with normal animals. BILSKI's conclusions are not very definite and do not quite coincide with what is said in the article itself. This is because Rana fusca is a difficult animal for experiments. Breeding to metamorphosis goes well, but there is then a great mortability also with control animals.

In later investigations (1926) with the same experiment animals, BILSKI finds that slight alcoholisation causes increased activity of the sex cells, heavy alcoholisation acts paralytically. His experiments have special significance with regard to the influence on male sex cells. It is expressed in the number and mortality of the larvae.

Frog larvae of alcoholised fathers have less tolerance against the action of alcohol than that of control material; movements f.i. sooner stop. Also the power of regeneration is smaller. It is remarkable that this difference disappears if the sex cells of alcoholised males after alcoholisation are placed in pure water for some time; the germ plasm was therefore not permanently injured.

In an experiment of heavy alcoholisation of male frogs the number of fertilizations is small, the larvae are smaller than with control material and the metamorphosis is retarded. After metamorphosis the young individuals are larger. The large number of fertilizations in case of slightly alcoholised material is ascribed by BILSKI to the influence on the mechanism of fertilisation. Alcohol in small quantities increases activity according to BILSKI; through the greater motility of the male gametes there are more fertilizations. In large quantities it has a paralytic effect on the living cells. BILSKI's results differ from those of HERTWIG (page 82).

BILSKI concludes from his experiments that alcoholisation of the germ-cells influences the mechanism of the fertilization and that moreover the germ plasm is injured; there is therefore a blastophthoric effect. It is a colloid chemical effect that does not lead to hereditary changes.

With regard to the parental alcoholism with men, BILSKI presumes that in consequence of the exciting effects on the germ cells more germcells take part in the fertilization; amongst which are also the weak germcells and the latter give an inferior progeny. We must accept here the fact, that apart from this the blasthopthoric effect makes itself felt. The hypothesis of BILSKI in his experiments is only weakly founded.

Summary and Conclusions

It is difficult to summarise the results of the different investigators in the experimental line. These experiments are only partly comparable. The quantity of alcohol which is given and the method of application are surely of signification for the result.

Another great difficulty is to get fully comparable control material. Material of the same hereditary properties for experiments and control is difficult to obtain; the outward circumstances likewise are not absolutely the same, and there is still the individual non-hereditary variability.

The requirements lead to inbreeding of the material, which we should like to avoid. It is therefore highly necessary for the experiments to be carried out under the most favourable conditions possible, for a long time and on a large scale, and they must be repeated with the same species of animals for different material.

It is also necessary to conduct the experiments with a view to finding out the influence of alcohol itself. The conditions can be made then as simple as possible. In this respect the experiments made by STOCKARD, PEARL, MACDOWELL, DANFORTH and others are at a disadvantage. During the investigation they had in view the problem of the heredity of acquired characteristics.

We now come to the following summary:

1. *The weight of treated animals.* Guinea pigs treated with subcutaneous injections of alcohol lose weight (FERRARI 1910). White mice become heavier (first experiment by NICE, 1912); they become lighter (second and third experiment by Nice, 1913, 1915).

STOCKARD's guinea pigs remain in a good condition with the inhalation method, emaciate if alcohol is administered through the mouth (1918 p. 140). The mortality in the first instance is not greater than that of control animals. PEARL's fowls (1916) become somewhat heavier, respiration is somewhat slower. DANFORTH's fowls (1919) decline in weight. ARLITT's and WELL's (1917) rats grew slower than control animals. MACDOWELL's (1921) white rats decline in weight. Albino rats (HANSON 1923) did not change in weight. Albino rats (HANSON and HEYS' 1924) declined in weight.
Through use of alcohol the body weight of experiment animals often declines. The inhalation method is less injurious than administration through the mouth.

2. *The fertility and the offspring of treated animals.*

a. Alcohol acts injuriously on the spermatozoids of the bull (KÖLLIKER). GÜNTHER finds a less injurious effect on dogs. IVANOW finds great resistability of spermatozoids in mammals. O. HERTWIG finds such a case of Rana after remaining in a solution of alcohol.

Spermatozoids therefore show a rather strong power of resistance when placed in a weak solution of alcohol. There are not many investigations on this point.

b. Very little is known of the resistance of non-fertilized egg-cells against alcohol (BILSKI).

c. α. The number of fertilizations. Alcoholisation of the fly Drosophila brings about a large and good progeny (MANN).

Frogs slightly alcoholized produce large and vigorous progeny. Strong alcoholisation causes paralysis of the gametes and gives small progeny. With these experiments there is a great individual variability (BILSKI 1921, 1926).

The fertility decreases in the experiments with fowls by CENI (1905).

The sexual sensitiveness in PEARL's fowls was increased immediately upon alcoholic inhalation. The number of infertile eggs in matings if the cock only is alcoholized shows no changes; if both parents are alcoholized the number of infertile eggs is very great. VAN DER HOEVEN in experimenting with fowls finds a large number of infertile eggs.

A third experiment by DANFORTH with heavy alcoholization of fowls shows a great many infertile eggs. FERRARI reports great infertility with guinea pigs. In the experiments made by LAITINEN with rabbits and guinea pigs there is great fertility. There is also great fertility in NICE's experiments with white mice; there are a large number of litters and the litters are also large.

BLUHM (1908) finds impotency with alcoholic male rats. When heavily alcoholizing white rats there is infertility, consequently a small number of litters and small litters. KOSTITSCH (1922) finds sterility with alcoholized white rats.

COLE and DAVIS find in their experiments with rabbits a smaller number of fertilizations. There is a considerable number of unsuccessful matings with STOCKARD's guinea pigs and a reduced propagative power.

The fecundity of alcoholized mice of ROMEIS' (comm. by BILSKI) is greater than of control animals.

In MAC DOWELLS experiments the number of litters was smaller with treated rats of the first generation. The size of litters was smaller. The fertility of treated albino rats of HANSON and HANDY is very low. One treated female proved to be a somewhat better breeder than the average control animal. It produced the whole alcoholic progeny.

From the different experiments it appears that the fertility i.e. the number of successful matings is sometimes lower and sometimes higher. There is certainly also an individual variability here and further the alcohol dosage will also have its significance.

c. β. *The developing germ* (see also 3). When alcoholizing the seeds of the melon, cucuma melo, PEARL (1926) in his experiments finds a lower germ percentage. Of the fertile eggs of the butterfly Selenia, which were heavily alcoholised, the mortality is enormous (HARRISON). The development of the frog becomes retarded (LAITINEN 1926). The development of treated fowls' eggs becomes retarded; fewer normal chickens are born (FÉRÉ).

MIRTO, who made similar experiments to those of FÉRÉ, found no difference with control eggs. Eggs of treated fowls give a smaller number of normal embryos (CENI).

In the case of PEARL's fowls, if both parents are alcoholized, the death rate before birth (prenatal) is small. In VAN DER HOEVEN's experiments there are a large number of prenatal deaths. Also in DANFORTH's third experiment the prenatal mortality is great.

Alcoholized eggs by PEARL show a great prenatal mortality in case of strong alcoholization.

There is a great prenatal mortality with STOCKARD's guinea pigs.

Albino rats of HANSON and HANDY show the fertility to be impaired. Three females (dams) were rendered completely sterile. One alcoholic female produced all the young which carried on the alcoholic line.

There were many prenatal deaths in the experiments with dogs by MAIRET and COMBEMALE.

The death rate before birth has been found to be very high in the experiments made by almost all investigators. Only in a few cases the mortality is small (experiments by PEARL with fowls where both parents were alcoholised, and in one case of the treated female albinorats in the experiment by HANSON and HANDY).

3. *The condition of the offspring* (see also 2). The seedlings (plants) of alcoholized seeds of cucuma melo mentioned in PEARL's experiments grow better than control material.

The condition of the few survivors in the experiments with Selenio by HARRISON is very good; they produce a healthy new stock.

In CENI's experiments the small number of chickens born is weak; there is a great mortality and the survivors are weak animals.

In PEARL's experiments with fowls the chickens do not differ from non-treated material if the cock only is alcoholized; if both parents have been treated the weight of young at birth is good and in growth they remain in advance of control material. The small number of chickens which came out in VAN DER HOEVEN's experiments are small weak, and sickly; there was great mortality.

Of eggs strongly alcoholized by PEARL only few hatched; furthermore a large number of this group died. In LAITINEN's experiments with rabbits and guinea pigs the offspring have a small body weight and remains backward in growth. There is a great mortality.

The condition of young pups in the experiments of MAIRET and COMBEMALE is bad, the mortality great. There is lack of vitality; epilepsy, tuberculosis and backwardness occur. PFÖRRINGER (1912) had the same results.

KERN (1910) finds among the offspring of treated guinea pigs a reduced resistance against tuberculosis and a great infant mortality. The offspring of BOURNÉVILLE's alcoholized guinea pigs all died of convulsions within some weeks.

Experiments with dogs in order to secure by alcoholic treatment offspring suffering from epilepsy had a negative result (BRATZ and HEBOLD).

BLUHM finds reduced fertility among the young of alcoholized rats.

The young of white mice of NICE's grow better in the first experiment; in the third the growth is irregular.

The young of white mice in AGNES BLUHM's experiments are frequently dead and develop badly. As an exception and in small litters vigorous animals sometimes occur.

The physical condition of STOCKARD's young of guinea pigs was unfavourable and growth remained retarded. The state of large litters is very bad. The survivors are irritable and nervous (1910—1915). On the other hand, the survivors are almost or quite as good as non-treated animals (1916—1917; 1919—1921).

The young of ARLITT and WELL's white rats are smaller. They show a marked lesser aptitude for learning.

The data about growth in MAC DOWELL's material are uncertain.

ROST and WOLF (1926) find in the case of rabbits no influence on the offspring.

Offspring of alcoholized male frogs are less resistent against alcoholization than control material (BILSKI, 1926).

The results about the conditions of the young do not correspond. Beside many experiments where the young are in a bad condition there are some where this is not the case. Sometimes well developed animals are met with beside many defective in the same experiment. The alcohol dosage and the individual variability probably explain this.

4. *The occurrence of monstra* in the alcohol experiments is certainly not general. FÉRÉ, who conducted so many experiments with fowls eggs, using all kinds of agents, found some. PEARL working in an entirely different manner, did not find any in alcoholized fowls.

In STOCKARD's alcohol material of guinea pigs there are a large number of monstrosities. Other investigators who also experimented with guinea pigs did not find any (BOURNEVILLE, FERRARI, KERN).

We may have before us here an instance of the uncertainty of the results of these experiments. It may be that STOCKARD worked with a special stock (although he occasionally added new animals to his material), it may also be that the outward circumstances were especially favourable for the appearance of monstra. Also R. GOLD-SCHMIDT reports on the great inconstancy of the results with his Drosophila tests at high temperatures (1929).

5. *Condition of the offspring in the successive generations.*

In MAIRET and COMBEMALE's experiments (1899) with dogs the young of the second generation are shown to be especially bad.

SCHRÖDER in his tests with rabbits in 6 generations finds great morbidity, mortality and small progeny. Some litters were well developed.

As an example of constitutional inferiority of the offspring (BLUHM) finds decreased fecundity of the young of alcoholized male rats.

In experiments on guinea pigs during 20 years, LAITINEN (1926) comes to the conclusion that alcohol in small quantities has a detrimental effect on the progeny, and which continues in several generations.

NICE finds in the second, as well as in the first, treated generations greater mortality among the young than among those of control material; it was, however, not greater than in the first generation. The fertility is also greater; there is a larger number of litters and the litters themselves are larger.

STOCKARD (1922) concludes from his material that the unfavour-able effects in the succeeding generations and by mating with non-treated material gradually become smaller. Finally, in the 4th generation the condition of the experimental material is slightly better than with control material.

In the experimenting years from 1910 to 1915 an increasing degeneracy of STOCKARD's alcoholized material is shown, there being a large number of malformations. In the 6th and 7th year of his ex-periments STOCKARD treated in an experiment males with alcohol for one and two generations against treating females for one and two generations. The results may be considered as supplying evidence of the increased effect of highe or longer alcohol dosage.

The intelligence of rats whose grandparents were treated with al-coholic fumes is somewhat inferior to that of control material (MACDOWELL and VICARI).

MacDowell finds the size of litters smaller in the following generations. The number of litters, which is smaller in the first generation, he finds with animals of treated parents and of treated grand-parents higher than of control material.

Treating the young with alcohol inhalation as compared with non-treated young of treated parents, does not appear to increase the defects with regard to control material.

Hanson thinks that in his material of albino rats the fertility which had suffered very much in the first two generations recovered gradually in later generations.

Hanson and Heys (1927) reporting on the results of their continued study of the resistance of the albino rat to alcoholic fumes in the course of ten generations, find that the animals during their lifetime gained some resistance against alcohol. Consequently they investigated further to see if this resistance to alcohol was already present at birth after ten generations. They then found the resistance to alcohol to be somewhat smaller and not greater. This points to blastophthory. Bilski (1926) experienced the same with frogs (page 103).

The results of the experiments about the significance of parental alcoholism for later generations are in general still indefinite. The experiments have not been conducted systematically. It appears that individual variability also occurs here (Schröder).

From the whole review of the experimental investigations we conclude that injury to the germ is brought about by alcohol. The result is injury to the germ cells and to the germ which makes itself felt on the developing germs and on the new born during growth. This is the general influence and is probably a phaenotypical phenomenon (false heredity). As a special result we find beside great mortality, the survival of some very resistable germs which appear to become vigourous individuals (alcohol proof).

We call the germ injury caused by alcohol a probable phaenotypical phenomenon, because it does not appear that the germ mass is permanently injured. The hereditary factors, the genes (the genotype) are not changed.

If we compare the value of the animal experiments with that of the observations with man for our knowledge of parental alcoholism, then we cannot place the value of animal experiments higher than that of the observations with man. Both methods of investigation have their limits and we must use both.

SMITH from Copenhague in collaboration with JOHANNSEN (1925) in his article about heredity and alcohol comes to the conclusion that "it cannot be considered as proved that by alcoholizing the genitor (animal or man), hereditary injury of the offspring occurs, and that it must be taken as improbable that such things will occur. The occurrence of changes in the conditions to the offspring in the first or the first successive generations on the basis of non-hereditary changes in the sex cells of the genitor are perhaps more probable, and in the experimental investigations of some investigators facts have been found which perhaps in some respect would point to this, but final, definite results are no more available here".

We can agree with the first part of the conclusions. The experience with alcohol used by man and in experiments with animals has not taught us anything about heredity of acquired characteristics. We must wait what the future will bring us in this respect (GUYER, H. J. MÜLLER, R. GOLDSCHMIDT).

Regarding the non-hereditary changes these may be doubted for so far as it will never be possible to fully exclude the fact that they do not arise from the hereditary characteristics of the families concerned or the experiment material.

From the review which has been given here, I think, however, that the standpoint of SMITH and JOHANNSEN may not be adopted and this must not be the last word about the effect of alcohol as a germ poison. The present day theoretical views repudiate to some extent the appreciation of parental alcoholism (page 76).

The whole material of facts about the significance of the use of alcohol by the parents for the children, the pathological anatomical investigation of the sex glands, the observations made with man as well as the experiments cause us to conclude that there is heredity and that there is germ injury. The injurious effects on the germs by alcohol does not spread to all germ cells. Some resistent germ cells occur. It would be incorrect to generalise from the fact that resistent germ cells occur, that alcohol acts as a selective agent. Most facts speak for the injurious influence of alcohol on the germ-

It is desirable that observations with man and experimental in. vestigations about parent alalcoholism are continued (see also p. 144).

B. THE OTHER GERM POISONS

1. Lead

TANQUEREL DES PLANCHES (1839) reports that some physicians of the last century saw the occurrence of amenorrhoe and even sterility in conjunction with lead colic. TANQUEREL himself did not meet with such things. He describes reduced potency with encephalopathy through lead poisoning (saturnism). Alcoholic abuse makes the illness much worse.

TANQUEREL reports further that animals living at large lead factories are impeded in their generative power; fowls stop laying.

The injurious effect on the progeny of persons who in the course of daily labour are exposed to lead poisoning has been thoroughly investigated by CONSTANTIN PAUL (1860) in a statistical arrangement of a very large material. The effect is most to be seen with female workers, but PAUL is of the opinion that the influence of the lead which is transmitted by the father to the child is also definite. There were 32 cases of pregnancy among 7 women by men showing signs of lead poisoning in the course of some years. Of these 11 cases lead to abortus. One child was still born. Of the 20 of those born alive 8 died in the first year, 4 in the second, 5 in the 3rd year, and only one grew up to be an adult. (PINARD cit. ROGER 1922; ROQUE 1872, cit. DÉJÉ-RINE; RENNERT, 1881, cit. LENZ, also report similar occurrences).

The influence of poisoned germ-cells of the father on the embryo must be viewed in the light of O. HERTWIG's investigations (see p. 137).

Abortions, still born and non-viable offspring are the most prevelant results of saturnism of the parents (ROGER 1922, REID, THOMPSON 1914, RUDEAUX 1910). KUFUSHIRO (1929) studied the pathological changes of ovary.

LEGRAND and WINTER (1889) report a case of both parents suffer-

ing from chronic lead poisoning. The father, a typographer, suffering from lead poisoning, was also somewhat inclined to drink; but
not so the mother. No lues. The woman was pregnant six times;
there was abortus three times during the first three months of pregnancy; one child was born at 7 months and succumbed two months
after birth, one child fully developed was born and died 7 months
later. The sixth time an eight months' child was born. The child was
thin and died 14 days after birth. At the post-mortem examination
nothing special was found.

Sir Thomas Oliver (1911) reported an epidemy of stillbirths in a
Yorkshire town, the cause of which was found to be drinking water
which had become contaminated by lead. With the removal of the
cause the effect ceased.

Since 1893 many cases have been reported from the midland
counties of England in which lead poisoning resulted from the use of
diachylon pills taken as an abortificient or in the belief that it might
act as a preventive (Witthaus 1911). As Paracelsus (cit. Roger
1922) wrote, the ancients possessed "des ceintures anaphrodisiaques"
of lead. Lieutard prescribed lead acetate for nymphomanie.

Porak, Pouchet and Meillère (cit. Roger) found lead in the
placenta and in the foetus. Lead is found back again in the milk of
goats, but in only very small quantities, and then after a lengthy
continued use of comparatively large quantities of lead acetate
(Koldewyn 1910).

It seems that not all individuals are susceptible to lead poisoning.
Jorès (1902) experimented with rabbits; the animals became very
thin, less active and became anaemic; the mortality is great. Animals
which survived gained in weight later (see also Stieglitz 1892).

In cases of heriditary saturnism Roger is of the opinion that the
possibility of syphilis and alcoholism of the parents must be thorough
ly investigated. Roger (1922) thinks that especially alcoholism of the
parents which so often occurs together with lead poisoning, favours
the influence of lead on the organism (Tanquerel, p. 112). Oliver
(1911) stated that a sexual idiosyncrasy in lead poisoning cannot be
ignored.

The result of investigations as to the health conditions of the
children in districts where workmen are exposed varies. Oliver
reports that in Staffordshire the surviving children of lead workers

Frets, Alcohol   8 are physically inferior to other children. They suffer from marasmus and have not the average vital stamina. The children of lead poisoned potters do not grow up into capable men and women like other children, but they are handicapped in their start of life, and subsequently many of them exhibit signs of mental as well as physical deterioration.

From the tables of the report of a commission of research, however it does not appear that working with lead has any injurious influence in lowering the birth rate, nor is there any evidence to show that the children of lead workers are any less healthy than those born of non-lead workers. (cf. GOADBY).

Quite different are the experiences in Hungary which country OLIVER himself visited. CHYZZER reports upon the conditions in the home potteries there. In some villages he found practically no children, while the inferior physical and mental development of the offspring of these pottery workers led him to conclude that infantilism, idiocy, and mental weakness were some of the effects of inherited plumbism. Deaths from hydrocephalus, acute meningitis, and convulsions were frequently noted among these children (cit. WELLER).

RUDEAUX states that of 442 pregnancies among the wives of lead workers there were 66 abortions and 241 miscarriages.

GOADBY concludes that there is little evidence for supposing that a male leadworker is less likely to beget children or that his children are more likely to be more unhealthy than those of men working in any other industrial process, provided that modern methods are employed to prevent absorption; and he adds: "In the absence of any precautions whatever as to daily absorption of dangerous dust, the effect on the offspring even in the case of male leadworkers, maty well be evident (cit. WELLER).

According to OPPENHEIM (1908), HARTMANN and DI GASPERO (1914), MARBURG (1919) chronic lead poisoning of the parents may cause epilepsy among the offspring. BUMKE (1924) reports that abortus is the most prevelant thing in the case of lead or mercury poisoning and that moreover, the children that survive appear to be weak and often predisposed to suffer from nervous diseases.

ANKER (1894, see also OPPENHEIM 1908) mentions a case of paralysis of the extensor muscles of the hands and the feet probably caused by saturnismus of the father. The child was imbecile (mother was healthy; 3 cases of abortus, sister healthy). OPPENHEIM (1908) mentions from the literature the report of BERGER that children of leadworkers not infrequently succumb to epilepsy. LEGRAND, ROQUE and SEELIGMULLER observed also other neuroses and organic diseases of the central nervous system

In the cases of acute lead poisoning ZINN (1899) mentions genital hemorrhagies and abortus. This apparently is due to the effect of lead poisoning on the muscle wall of the uterus (see below). BAADER (1928) in an article on lead-poisoning says that lead acts preferably on the elements of the blood, on the muscles (especially of the blood vessels of the intestines and uterus), and on the perifere and central nervous system.

The experimental evidence of a blastophthoric effect of lead poisoning is the following. FÉRÉ (1893) in experimenting with injections of active substances on fowls eggs (p. 80), also used a solution of lead nitrate. He brought about a retardation of the development and the formation of monstrosities.

ANNINO (1894) found as a result of his extensive experimental studies of rabbits to which lead was administered in the food, that the development of embryos was interrupted.

In the case of fowls eggs incubated after painting the shell over with a strong solution of lime and others with a solution of lead nitrate, OLIVER (1911) found that while all the eggs painted with lime came to maturity, those painted with lead nitrate did not produce one single living chick. Upon opening the latter eggs the embryo was always found to have reached a fair stage of development. Similarly in the case of pregnant rabbits to whom lead was administered in food, miscarriage took place. Pregnant guinea pigs confined in hutches lined with paper found to contain lead aborted (CHARRON). All the pregnant animals which were given lead aborted. These experimental results confirm the abortificient action of diachylon (p. 113; LEGGE and GOADBY, GLIBERT). ROGER (1922, p. 116) reports similar results with the lead experiments made by ROBERT, BALLAND, POUCHET, PORAK. ROBERT thinks that lead brings about a contraction of the muscles, which would explain the sensitivity of the uterus in respect to abortions.

COLE and BACHHUBER (1914) report experiments with lead in the form of lead acetate. The method of double mating practised by

COLE and DAVIS (p. 85) was employed. They found that the off-spring produced by male rabbits, which have been poisoned by injecting lead acetate into the alimentary tract, have a lower vitality and are distinctly smaller in average size than normal offspring of unpoisoned males.

Similar results were obtained with fowls. Normal hens were mated with a cock which was fed daily with a certain quantity of lead aceta-te. Of the 174 eggs laid by normal hens mated with a treated cock 47 were infertile (27 %) and 35 embryos died in shell (27.5 %), 92 chicks hatched, 13 dying within 3 weeks (14.1 %). Control matings produced 42.3 % infertile eggs, 17.2 % embryos died in shell and 37 % died in 3 weeks time.

In this experiment there is a very high percentage of infertile eggs of control matings (PEARL 1917, p. 250, also remarks on this). The percentage of deaths of embryos in shell is low and as low the percentage for chicks which died in 3 weeks (see page 88). Of the 4 matings with the treated cock the figures differ greatly.

In the second experiment three white Leghorn hens were coupled alternately with a treated Leghorn cock and with a normal Houdan cock. There were 109 eggs, 46 (42.1 %) of which were infertile, i.e. the same percentage as for control matings in the first experiment. Seventeen embryos died, 10 of which could be identified (9 Leghorns and 1 crossbred), 46 chicks hatched, 31 being Leghorns and 15 cross-breds; 5 Leghorns died within 3 weeks but no crossbreds.

In the experiments of COLE and BACHHUBER with alternate breed-ing, the number of matings with treated male is not smaller than with normal male as in the alcohol test by COLE and DAVIS. The con-ditions are not alike, because the normal male is of another variety.

Of the 63 fertile eggs, 17 embryos died in the shell, namely 27 %, the same percentage as for matings with the lead male in the first experiment. Of the 31 lead chickens hatched 5 died, in three weeks, i.e. 16.1 % the same percentage as for matings with the lead male in the first experiment and more than for control matings. Of the 15 cross-bred (control) chicks not one died within three weeks.

In both experiments of COLE and BACHHUBER the results of the matings of a normal female and a treated male are more unfavour-able than the matings of a normal female and a normal male. The large number of infertile eggs in the control matings of the first experiment makes the significance of the control material uncertain.

In these experiments we have a fine example of the study of blastophthory because only the male animal was poisoned.

WELLER (1915) gave guinea pigs repeated weighed doses (5—80 milligrammes) of commercial white lead in capsules through the mouth. The doses were so small and the frequency such as not to interfere with the alimentation of the experimental animals.

These guinea pigs were mated; lead males with normal females and further lead females with normal males. Control matings were made and the normal females were also mated alternately with lead males and with normal males. A total of 93 matings yielded 170 young.

Of 34 matings of lead males with normal females 65 young were produced with an average birth weight of only 66.3 grm. Of 27 matings of normal male and lead females there were 47 young with an average weight of 69.3 grm. (control young weighed 81.5 grms.) Twelve young of lead males and 8 young of lead females were still born or died in the first week against 5 young of control parents. Of the three stunted descendants of a lead father the smallest died on the fourth day but the other two grew to maturity in spite of the fact that they were but little more than half the normal size at birth.

There is some irregularity in the results. In several instances lead poisoned males failed for two or three months to impregnate any of the females with which they were running. The average number of offspring per mating of the treated males is practically the same as in the group of normal pigs. Only one treated male proved to be completely sterile. The offspring of a treated parent which are decidedly below the average weight at birth remain permanently under weight as compared with control pigs of the same age. Lead poisoned females have many stillborn. Besides the reduced natal weight, great mortality during the first few days after birth was the most striking change shown by the offspring of the lead poisoned males. In only two instances were malformations observed in the first filial generation.

An apparent recovery of the germ plasm takes place some time after the administration of lead has been stopped. This point requires to be investigated further.

Summary. Saturnism of the father gives corresponding deviations with the offspring as saturnism of the mother. We know by observations with man and by experiments with animals that lead has an injurious action on the offspring. We find sterility in women, reduced potency in the man. Abortions, still-born and non-viable embryos, defective children among whom there is epilepsy.

Simultaneous alcoholism increases the occurrence of the symptoms of saturnism. Saturnism with the father produces the same defects in the offspring as that of the mother. There is a varying disposition for lead poisoning.

From the experiments with animals it is also shown that the condition of the young of treated animals is more unfavourable than with control animals, also if the male alone is treated these disadvantages are found in the offspring. If no further lead is given to the parents, the inferiority of the offspring in the successive litters soon ceases. The results of the experiments do not yet allow the expression of any opinion about other detail.

2. Mercury

Very little is mentioned in the literature of mercury being significant as a germ poison.

BUMKE (1924, page 16) states that abortus is most frequent as a result of mercury (KUSSMAUL) or lead poisoning and that the surviving children are weak and nervous. GOETZ and SCHAULL have both noticed a case of congenital tremor in children of mercury poisoned female factory labourers. (ROGER 1922). KUSSMAUL (1861) describes a case of malformation with a daughter of a patient suffering from mercurialism (p. 158). He further states (p. 328, 233) that with these patients irregular menstruation occurs, and that pregnancy would lead to abortion and premature birth. The children are often weak. LEWIN (1899) reports of women in Memel in Lithuania swallowing metallic quicksilver pre par ed as a kind of grey ointment, as a medium of abortification. According to KOLDEWIJN quicksilver does not go over into the milk. The literature in general is not very extensive (KULKOW 1928).

As to experiments with animals, GASPARD (1821) exposed fowls eggs to mercury vapour in an incubator and saw the embryos die very early, even before blood formation (cit. DARESTE and FÉRÉ). DARESTE

(1893) repeated the experiments, and in contrast to GASPARD found that quicksilver does not hinder the development of the embryos. FÉRÉ (1894) conducted his experiments in the manner already explained (page 80). He laid the eggs in a space full of quicksilver vapour for some time and then placed them in a thermostat for the development of the embryo. Of 29 control eggs eight were infertile; there were two monstrosities and nineteen normal embryos of about 44. Of 29 treated eggs seven are infertile; there are seven malformations and 15 normal embryos of 36 hours. There is therefore a slightly retarding influence on the development and likewise a slight teratogene influence.

KOELLIKER (1856) points out that QUATREFAGES was the first to show that metal salts are not absolutely harmful to mammals, yet for each kind of salt there must be a certain dilution in order to prevent it from having any detrimental action. KOELLIKER found in the case of mercury chloride dissolved in a sugar solution 1 : 10.000 and added to the spermatozoids of a bull, and which otherwise would act very favourably, had no effect at all.

Summary. Nothing much is known of quicksilver as a germ poison.

3. Thallium

As a medicine thallium was given for some time to sufferers from lung trouble, because of its antihydrotic action on night sweating. Thallium stands in the sixth period between mercury and lead. In its trivalent form it has no action; in its monovalent form it causes impediment to growth and feeding, and causes the hair to fall out.

By way of experiment BUSCHKE and PEISER (1922) find that when fed with thallium, rats did not grow so well and that with adults the sexual instinct disappears. In three cases when dissecting they found complete atrophy of the testicles so much so that macroscopically there was no testicle substance to be seen. HECKE (1928) gave rats and rabbits thallium acetium on bread. In the case of acute poisoning there was macroscopically no change to be seen in the organs, and also histologically, changes were hardly to be expected (page 9). HECKE therefore gave small quantities to his test animals daily in order to obtain a slow action. In the experiments described by HECKE with the rats the poison was injected subcutaneously and sometimes given through the mouth. Upon histological examination of the testicles he found great changes to the spermatozoids and in the various preliminary stages, and he considers disturbance in the power of propagation highly probable. There is great diversity in the individual sensitiveness.

According to BUSCHKE and BERMANN (1927) rutting with mice stops if thallium, lead, and arsenic (partly) are given. BUSCHKE and PEISER remark that although the desire for sexual intercourse is reduced, yet now and then cases of pregnancy occur. The use of thallium causes the hair to fall out, as has been stated before. These investigators found in their experiments with young alopexie of a congenital nature.

Summary. The experiments with thallium are important. With males a reduction of libido sexualis is found, and with regard to pathologic-anatomical changes, atrophy of the testicles. There is great variability of individual sensitiveness.

4. Arsenic and Antimony

According to BLOEMENDAL (1908) arsenic does not go over into the blood circulation of the foetus. He gave a rabbit from the beginning of pregnancy 12 mg. $As_2 O_3$ daily. The animal bore seven normal young. One of them which was examined showed no traces of arsenic. In another experiment arsenic pure was given. The same animal bore nine dead animals. Two of the animals were examined, but there were no traces of arsenic. BROUARDEL (1902). examined the foetus of a pregnant woman who had died from tuberculosis and who had been treated with arsenic preparations, but no arsenic was found. In a solution of Kal. arsenicosum 1 : 1000 spermatozoids after 3 minutes stop all movement. (GÜNTHER 1907). HEFFTER and KEESER (1927) report on experiments with $As_2 O_3$. The young were larger and heavier, but were all stillborn. KOSTITCH and VERBITZKI (1927) give liquor Fowleri in the food of male white rats (1—2 mg p. die; 1—4 months). The animals are in a good condition, the bodyweight increases, but the post mortem examination of the testicles shows changes, that KOSTITCH already found in his experiments with alcohol (p. 97) and with jodine (p. 122). The various stages of development of the spermatozoids disappear in inversed succession; at last there is azoospermia.

The influence on the metabolism which expresses itself by an increase of weight of body is mentioned repeatedly. FOKKER contests this (CROCE 1911, FOKKER 1872).

HODGSON (1927) injected 44 white mice with 0.01 grms. organic antimony compound on alternate days. The results ended in a failure to conceive, to abortus, injury to the foetus or to all three.

Summary. Observations with man about the action of arsenic as a germ poison are not to be found in the literature. Experimentally arsenic has a highly intoxicating effect on the spermatozoids and on the foetus; so has antimony.

5. Phosphor

I have not found any observation in the literature about the action of phosphor as a germ poison. In the manuals about toxicology in general very little is said of poisons as germ poisons. Phosphor passes into the blood (HARTMANN, LEMKES 1916). Phosphor fumes penetrate through the shell of eggs and create monstrosities and general retardation of the development. (FÉRÉ 1895). YAMANE and KATO (1928) investigated the influence of a solution of dextrose phosphate ($^1/_{10}$ norm $Na_2 HP O_4$ plus $^1/_{10}$ norm. $Na H_2PO_4$ and 4 % dextrose) on the spermatozoids of rabbits.

6. Iodine

When FÉRÉ (1899) subjected fowls eggs for some time to an iodine atmosphere and afterwards placed them in a thermostat, his results varied according to the position of the eggs. Where the germ was facing upwards there were many malformations; if the germ rested on the bottom the development was normal because then the fumes had not reached the germ. By injecting a solution of an iodine combination into the developing fowls eggs, the development is somewhat retarded; it continues however and there is no mortality. There is great tolerance for iodine combinations. The same quantity kitchen salt solution of a same percentage is more harmful. If iodine combinations cause abortus, this, according to FÉRÉ, is not caused by their action on the embryo. Similar results were obtained when injecting with bromide. It is not to be wondered at that pregnant women who use 20 grammes of potassium experience no difficulties in respect to the pregnancy. See also MAC DOUGAL (page 137) and FLEIG (p. 124).

LOEB and ZOPPRITZ (1918) gave salts of iodine to white mice in the food. Pregnant animals aborted. The animals, both male and female, became sterile. After stopping administration of iodine, fertility returns after one month. The doses causing sterility are below the toxic working, i.e. health and alimentation are not perceptibly affected.

ADLER (1914) undertook experiments with the larvae of salamanders and with guinea pigs and rabbits, using iodine albumen combinations. At first he found no anatomical changes in the germ glands of rabbits, whilst, however, a distinct sterility arose with the males as well as with the females. As explanation ADLER thought this to be due to action on the internal glands; he points out the frequency of sterility in those suffering from morbus BASEDOWI (lit. ADLER). When ADLER gave large doses of iodine he found distinct changes in the testicles. In these important investigations of 60 testicles they appear to be macroscopically atrophical, and microscopically, ADLER found that the sperm-forming cells were destroyed and the interstitial cells profilerated. These are changes following upon acute action, similar to those occurring after ray treatment. ADLER also finds a great difference in the individual sensitiveness; also in respect to the different canals of the same testicles. He did not find these changes when giving the animal potassium iodine. Then there were hardly ever any pregnancies, although there were, so to say, no changes in the testicles. ADLER reminds us of information of earlier authors who found changes in the testicles as a result of giving patients prolonged treatment with iodine potassium. (see also FÉRÉ).
In ADLER's opinion the molecular iodine is the most active part of the iodine combinations. KOSTITCH and TELEBAKOVITCH (1926) find degeneration of the sex cells of the testicles of white rats in their experiments with jodine.

Summary. According to more recent researches (ADLER, KOSTITCH) iodine is a germ poison. Earlier investigators (FÉRÉ 1890) found only a slight effect in this respect.

7. Nicotine

O. and R. HERTWIG (1887) placed unfertilized eggs of sea urchins for 5—15 minutes in seawater to which a drop of nicotine extract had been added. The later fertilisation is then effected; if a weak solution is used, not with all eggs; there are individual differences. Some of the eggs have a great power of resistance, others less so against harmful influences. There is polyspermy; there enter 2,3 and more spermatozoids in the egg, which unite in various numbers with the egg nucleus. Among the malformations which arise are more compact larvae, which HERTWIG calls stereoblastula. Fertilised eggs of the sea urchin (Echinoidea) are not impeded in their development by nicotine solution, but it is somewhat retarded. Spermatozoids of the seaurchin can withstand a stay in nicotine better than the eggs. For eggs O and R. HERTWIG took 1 drop of extract in 100, 200 tot 1000 ccm seawater, and for the spermatozoids the solution was 10 times stronger. After a stay of 15 minutes the spermatozoids are still very mobile (tumultuary movement). After 35 minutes they are still so. The power of fertilisation has not yet been disturbed. An hour later the spermatozoids are still fairly mobile; their pregnatory powers have suffered a little, but only temporarily; for when HERTWIG then placed these spermatozoids in contact with eggs in fresh seawater, fertilisation at first appeared not to take place; after a quarter of an hour, however, all eggs were normally pregnant. The spermatozoids have a great resistibility. G. and P. HERTWIG placed spermatozoids of the Rana esculenta in a weak solution of nicotine (0.15 and 0.25 %) for one hour. The spermatozoids maintained their mobility and accomplished fertilisation, whilst development of the eggs was also normal. G. and P. HERTWIG saw in such experiments also the revival of the movements, yet upon longer immersion the mobility became reduced and finally stiffness set in. When the authors diluted the solution with seawater, while the spermatozoids are very mobile, (in tumultuary movement) the spermatozoids became immobile. In these experiments a very poor state of fertilisation was obtained. G. and P. HERTWIG presume that the other results of O. and R. HERTWIG's experiments with sperm of sea urchins is to be attributed to the weak nicotine solution which they think was used by O. and R. HERTWIG (this solution was ten times stronger than that which they used for eggs; thus 1 drop of extract to 10 or 100 ccm. seawater; cf. O and R. HERTWIG 1887, page 4 and 43).

Crossing experiments with the spermatozoids of the Rana esculenta treated with nicotine with the eggs of Rana fusca did not produce any results and therefore proved that there was no partial destruc tion of the germ substance of the spermatozoids (G. and P. HERTWIG 1913).

Tobacco smoke and nicotine fumes injure fowls eggs. When placed later in the incubator very few develop. There is retardation of development and there are malformations (FÉRÉ). FÉRÉ (1895) also undertook an experiment by injecting a weak solution of nicotine into the albumen of the egg. Of the 46 eggs injected with water 33 developed into normal embryos, and of the 46 eggs with nicotine solution there were only 16 normal embryos. Remarkable in this respect is the fact that the development of the normal embryos in the nicotine group is more advanced than in the water group (Nicotine group average 73 hours, water group average 45.5 hours). The em- bryos which have resisted the toxic action of nicotine are therefore more developed than control embryos, says FÉRÉ. He also noticed something similar when using terpentine extract fumes. He connects this phenomen with the stimulatory action of some poisons given in small doses. We are also reminded here of PEARL's interpretation of his experiments with fowls (p. 87) and of the "arsenic proofness" mentioned by EHRLICH, The mobility of spermatozoids of a dog had not ceased after an immersion of nicotine 1 : 1000 after 93 minutes (GÜNTHER 1907).

RICHON and PERRIN (1908) find that young rabbits submitted to nicotine poison remain backward in growth and emaciate. If injec- tions are stopped the animals recover very quickly and completely. If guinea pigs are treated with tobacco fumes or with injections of iodi- ne (FLEIG 1908) all young are defective. They are still born, there is frequency of abortus and the weight of the survivors is very low. Their growth is slow and they do not live long. It is a great exception if an animal becomes an adult; the animals remain thin and stunted. NICE (1912, 1913) experimented with white mice giving them nico- tine and treating them with tobacco smoke during two generations (see also page 82). In both generations the mice that were subjected to tobacco smoke, bore more young than those of the other experi- ments (with alcohol and caffein), while the control animals had the lowest number of offspring. Tobacco smoke excercised a very marked injurious action on the viability of the young, seeing that 37 %

(41 : 111) of the first generation and 26 % (26 : 101) of the second generation died through lack of viability. In this group there was one miscarriage. Nicotine had not such a strong action. The control young grew roughly in the same proportion as those treated with nicotine and with smoke.

The offspring of nicotine poisoned parents to which no nicotine was given were somewhat heavier than the young which were given nicotine. The young subjected to smoke and those not subjected to such grew practically in the same proportion. In the first experiment all the mice increased in weight, in the 2nd experiment (1913) their growth was perhaps somewhat checked. Also in the case of these investigations by NICE about the action of nicotine, the young of the survivors of the test animals were not inferior to those of control animals (see page 84).

ROGER reporting on tobaccoism says that there is a tendency to abortion. FRIEDBERGER (1926) going on the basis of the experience that female tobacco workers have miscarriages very often, subjected rats to heavy cigar smoke. He found in the progeny no differences in respect to control animals. The experimental animals emaciate to 50% of the body weight says VON ZEBROWSKI. HATCHER and GROSBY (1928) found nicotine in the milk of a cigarets smoking mother.

HOFSTÄTTER (1923) undertook experiments with dogs, rabbits and rats by injecting nicotine. The experiments were interrupted owing to the war and have only a preliminary character. HOFSTÄTTER worked with large doses and obtained strong reactions. He reports about 9 dogs (7 females and two males) which he injected subcutaneously $\frac{1}{2}$—2 ccm of a 5 % solution of nicotinum tartaricum MERCK (100 parts nic. tart. is equal to 32.53 parts nicot. puriss.) The animals nearly always emaciate and have a reduced sexuality or this stops altogether. There are many cases of abortions with pregnant dogs and many still births. The surviving animals are in bad health and grow slowly. It is not quite certain if this is owing to the condition of the young themselves, because subcutaneous injections of nicotine were continually given to the mother during suckling, and nicotine was traced in the milk (see page 127).

Upon dissection of the test animals the different organs were shown to be very much changed. In the female animals the ovaries were atrophied and degenerated and in the males the testicles. The germ glands of the young animals were hypoplastic and showed fatty degeneration.

The results of the experiments with rabbits (11 does and two bucks) correspond with those with dogs. HOFSTÄTTER gave an injection of $\frac{1}{2}$—3 cm³, 1 % nicotine solution. The animals were mostly thin, upon dissection the ovaries were seen to be atrophied and degenerated and in most cases there were few matured follicles. He finds atrophy of the internal genital organs as found with powerful X-ray treatment. The testicles show atrophy and very much impaired spermatogenesis. The sexual desire ceases.

The pregnant animals have a frequency of abortions, there are many stillbirths and those alive are in a bad condition. Of the two surviving one died e.g. in 16 days, the other in 6 weeks. These animals were very much emaciated and showed signs of severe atrophy of all internal organs. The testicles were hypoplastic and as it would seem there is a condition of primary injury to the organs.

Rats are highly susceptible to nicotine. HOFSTÄTTER reports of 11 females and 2 males. He gave 0.5—1 ccm of a 1 % nicotine solution. The acute action is less, but the animals mostly die within a few weeks. The animals become very thin. Upon dissection atrophy of the ovaries was found. The testicles of males were in different stages of atrophy. The sexual instinct had disappeared. The second male survived the injections and pregnated a normal female three months later. This animal cast four young ones which died a few days later. Upon dissection nothing peculiar was found.

When experimenting with white mice in order to get a first impression of the fertility of nicotine poisoned mice HOFSTÄTTER found a greater mortality among the test animals than among control animals and the number of survivors was smaller. The difference in the results of HOFSTÄTTER's and NICE's experiments is especially to be attributed to the vastly different doses of nicotine poison. HOFSTÄTTER used mostly a 1 % solution of nicotine tartrate MERCK, gave 0.5 to 1 ccm per diem. To rabbits he gave up to 7 ccm in the food. NICE used a 1 % solution and mixed 2 ccm of same in the food. By this method it is uncertain how much of the poison is taken up by the mice. Yet NICE states that grey rats died in 9 days in this manner, whilst a solution of 1 : 500 was fatal for white mice.

Many investigators obtained the same results as HOFSTÄTTER. We cite still the following from HOFSTÄTTER's publication. Observations about changes to the testicles in man by the effects of nicotine do not appear to have been made.

S. WRIGHT experimenting with dogs gave them tobacco in the food and found a curtailment and stoppage of sexual instinct. The testicles were soft and small. G. PETIT gave dogs, fowls, guinea pigs and rabbits tobacco in the food and shut them up in a space into which smoke was let or administered a nicotine solution into the intestines. In the case of acute as well as in the case of chronic tobacco poisoning PETIT finds important changes in the testicles; in the last named cases he found interstitial atrophy and azoospermy. GY found no marked changes in rabbits. PERAZZI injected subcutaneously female rabbits with a tobacco macerate and often found in the ovaries degeneration and induration. The embryos in the uterus die and the growth of the young is distinctly worse than with control animals. Sterility in the mother animals occurs. PETIT also found the ovaries atrophic and indurated. R. MÜLLER found when experimenting with white mice and canaries strongly reduced libido and upon fertilisation many deaths and non-viable young. UNGER's results were not so marked in respect to germ injury.

The reduced potency of the man through nicotine poisoning and the reduced fertility of female tobacco workers are connected by HOFSTÄTTER in the experiences with experiments with animals.

NASSE, SUGIMOTO, FRÜHARP, ADLER and AYMERISCH investigated the action of nicotine administration on the muscles of the uterus in experiments with animals; the result varies. According to DIXON (HEFFTER 1927) nicotine affects the smooth muscular tissue and according to one experiment caused abortus in the case of a pregnant cat. WADDELL studied the pharmacology of the genital auxiliary organs.

AYMERISCH in his experiments with guinea pigs arrived at the following results. By slow poisoning brought about by rubbing in a nicotine unguent, no influence is noticed during the course of pregnancy, although nicotine can be traced in the maternal organs. The foetus dies as a result of nicotine injection. Nicotine does not go into the foetus in noticeable quantities.

HOFSTÄTTER's results differ from AYMERISCH's in respect to the last mentioned point. HOFSTÄTTER is of the opinion that nicotine passes through the placenta to the foetus and accepts the statement that nicotine passes from the mother into the child through the milk. He concludes in the animal experiments that as there are nearly always important changes to the testicles to be traced it is certain that these organs are seriously injured by nicotine.

Summary. Nicotine poisoning brings about a reduced potency in man, reduced fertility in women.

In the experiments with animals it has been found that spermatozoids of lower animals can resist the action of nicotine very well, whilst the eggs have less resistance. With frogs somewhat different results were obtained. Considerably smaller numbers of normal embryos were obtained with treated fowls eggs. Among the normal there were some very good ones. Of the mammals the sperm of the dog can stand immersion in a nicotine solution well.

The development of the embryos of mammals in the different experiments is varied. NICE finds principally great mortality. FLEIG finds great mortality and unhealthy condition of survivors. HOFSTÄTTER who administered large doses of nicotine found many abortions and still born among dogs. The surviving young are in a bad state. The pathological anatomical changes are considerable in the ovaries and testicles of the experimental animals. These changes are also evident with a few viable young of treated parents. The manifold abortions may be explained by the action of the smooth muscles of the uterus. Various other investigators also found pathological-anatomical modifications of the sexual glands. Also in the case of nicotine poisoning there is varying individual disposition.

8. Caffeine

FÉRÉ (1900) says that caffeine is one of those poisons which perhaps when injected into a fowl's egg in small quantities would act favourably on the development of the embryo and when administered in large quantities would act detrimentally.

He undertook the following experiments (table 12). In these experiments the great variability as to the percentage of monstrosities in control eggs is striking. Taking into account the variability it is also uncertain whether the great age of the embryos of treated eggs according to the degree of development, is really of significance in the fourth experiment.

NICE (1912, 1913) made his experiments with white mice also with caffein (page 82). See also VACCAS, and BLUHM (cit. BLUHM, 1930).

STIEVE (1928) reports on experiments with rabbits. When he gives male rabbits large doses of caffein for a short time, the young of most litters die within the first week after birth; females that received caffein before fertilization, show a great sterility and pregnant females show a great prenatal mortality. Especially of the first two experiments the young, that survive are in a good condition and they have later a normal offspring (see also FRETS, 1931).

Summary. There are some experiments with caffeine as a germ poison. The experiments by FÉRÉ as well as those by NICE are still uncertain in their results. The mortality of the offspring is great. The results of STIEVE are important; he finds a great blastopthorous effect of spermatozoids and eggcells.

TABLE 12. INJECTIONS OF FOWLS EGGS WITH A SOLUTION OF CAFFEIN. (FÉRÉ 1900). TREATED EGGS; INJECTED WITH COFFEIN.

N. of exp.	N. Series	N. eggs.	CC.	°/₀₀	m.g.	Incubation hours	Chickens						
							Norm.	%	age	infertile	%	monstra	%
1	4	48	0.75	16	12	72	4	8.3	48	6	12.5	38	79.2
2	6	72	0.5	16	8	72	45	62.5	45h.20	6	8.3	21	29.2
3	6	72	0.25	16	4	72	51	70.8	47h.27	5	6.9	16	22.2
4	6	72	0.2	10	2	72	48	66.7	51h.41	5	6.9	24	33.3

CONTROL EGGS; INJECTED WITH AQ. DEST.

N. of exp.	N. Series	N. eggs.	CC.	°/₀₀	m.g.	Incubation hours	Norm.	%	age	infertile	%	monstra	%
1	4	48	0.75			72	28	58.3	45h. 9	6	12.5	13	27.1
2	6	72	0.5			72	55	76.4	47h. 8	7	9.7	10	13.9
3	6	72	0.25			72	52	72.2	46h.27	1	1.4	18	25
4	6	72	0.2			72	49	68.1	49h.41	3	4.2	23	32

9. Morphine, Opium, Codeine, Cocaine, Hydras Chlorali

Morphine and opium are also mentioned as germ poisons, although clinical experience in connection with these is not available. (O. BINSWANGER 1899 page 84, FÉRÉ 1890 page 248).

Lengthy use of cocaine leads to sexual impotency (JOËL, 1923 also STROHMAYER, 1928).

KOELLIKER (1856) already undertook experiments with spermatozoids of a bull and others, using morphine. Motility ceased but returned after administration of 1 % solution of kitchen salt.

In their experiments connected with the action of chemical substances on non-fertilized eggs of the seaurchin, O. and R. HERTWIG (1887) found that morphine had only a slight influence. Only concentrated solutions (0.4—0.6 %) in not too long an action produced the same deviations in the later fructification as shown by the action of other poisons. Morphine in the usual solutions seems to have no effect on the spermatozoids of the sea urchin. Fertilized eggs of the sea urchin show also great indifference to morphine solutions.

FÉRÉ (1893) injected into fowls eggs small quantities of a morphine solution and placed them in an incubator. Development was retarded and there were monstrosities.

Codeine injected into fowls eggs also produces retardation of development and formation of monstrosities. (FÉRÉ 1893).

Cocaine injected into eggs of the seaurchin showed the same departures in eggs fertilised afterwards as did also different other substances which O. and R. HERTWIG (1887) investigated. It differs in its action somewhat from chloral hydrate (see below).

Fertilised eggs in their development are very much impeded by cocaine. In a solution of cocaine 1 : 1000 the spermatozoids of the dog do not stop their movement after 60 minutes immersion (GÜN-THER 1909). The same with a similar solution of morphine.

Hydrastine hydrochlorate has a deleterious effect on the eggs of the seaurchin. Upon later fertilisation divergencies occur which were pursued by O. and R. HERTWIG in vivo (1887). Hydrastine hydrochlorate acts on the spermatozoids of the sea urchin very drastically. The motility disappears, returns however after some time. Defects in the fertilised product were not found (O. and R. HERTWIG, 1887). The fertilisation of eggs of the sea urchin becomes disturbed by chloral solutions. Fertilised eggs are impeded very much in their development.

G. and P. HERTWIG (1913) could not find any injurious effect with the sea urchin. They also treated the spermatozoids of Rana Fusca with a $\frac{1}{2}$ % solution of chloral hydrate and had them fertilized with the eggs of Rana esculenta. Some cross breeds developed; a proof of part elimination of the spermachromatine (page 134).

O. HERTWIG (1913) placed spermatozoids of the frog, Rana Fusca, in a 0.3 % solution of hydras chlorali for half an hour and two hours respectively. Afterwards they were united with normal eggs. In the first experiment all the eggs were fertilised, in the second experiment only half of them. In both cases only pathologic larvae developed. Control eggs without exception developed into normal embryos. Among pathologic larvae there were some with spina bifida, many were too small, others succumbed. Development became slower. All chloral treated embryos are to be distinguished from non-treated by their dwarfed condition, they only being two thirds or half of the size of comparison animals. They do not move freely.

Diploide gametes and polyploidie (the occurrence of multiples with the number of chromosomes) may be formed by narcotica. (O. ROSENBERG, 1928).

Summary. There are hardly any observations with man as to the injurious effects of the poisons named under article 9. In the experiments hardly any action or only a slight influence of morphine was found. The action of cocaine is stronger and that of hydras chlorali is the strongest. The experiments with hydras chlorali with spermatozoids of Rana Fusca by O. HERTWIG and by G. and P. HERTWIG are fine examples of blastophthoric influences. However even here individual variability must be considered.

10. Alcohols (except Aethylalcohol), Glycerine, Dextrine, Chloroform, Aether and Acetone

Methylalcohol.

The results of inhalation experiments with methylalcohol with fowls by PEARL (1917) correspond greatly with those of similar experiments with aethylalcohol (page 87).

The treated fowls increase in weight. The laying of the birds has been excellent. There are many infertile eggs. There is a great difference in the results of the various matings. PEARL finds the following in three matings of methyl treated males and females.

mating	eggs set	infertile	% infertile	died inshell	% died in shell	hatched	% hatched
2120	34	32	94,1	1	50 %	1	50
2121	24	4	37,5	3	20 %	12	80
2122	27	26	96,3	0	0,0 %	1	100

We see in mating 2120 that 1 of 2 embryos died in the shell (50 %) and in mating 2122 there were no deaths with one embryo (0.0 %). Of these totals the mean figures are taken.

PEARL concludes that fertile eggs of treated animals hatch better than eggs of normal animals. The weight when hatched, the growth and the total surviving animals are better with the offspring of treated animals than with control animals. There were no deformities.

In solutions of methyl-, propyl-, isobutyl- amyl- and allylalcohol of 1 % the motility of dogs sperm which has been weakened by standing two hours, stops in about twenty minutes. In a solution of methylalcohol of 5 %, this time is 5 minutes for sperma of a bull, a very short time (GÜNTHER 1907).

FÉRÉ during his studies about teratogene influence of alcohols in the albumen of fowls eggs not only injected aethylalcohol but also methylalcohol, propyl-, butyl- and amylalcohol. The higher alcohols according to FÉRÉ show an increasing degree of harmfulness. Wine and especially brandy are more detrimental than pure alcohol. Absinthe and aniseed essences produce the greatest number of defects. The chickens which survived were often subject to epileptic fits (page 77).

Fowls eggs exposed some time to fumes of absinthe essence showed disturbance in their later development (FÉRÉ 1893).

GRÉHANT (1900) on the grounds of his experiments with absinthe and the investigations of the proportion of alcohol in the blood, thinks that essence of absinthe acts on the body by reason of the alcohol it contains (LABORDE and MAGNAN think the same, page 7).

Experiments with fowls eggs by injecting into the albumen teach us that methylalcohol has a stronger teratogenic influence than aethylalcohol but less than propylalcohol. In such experiments the teratogenic influence of the isoalcohols increases as well as that of the alcohols according to the ratio of CO_2. (FÉRÉ).

O. HERTWIG (1912) experimented with spermatozoids of the Rana using methyl- and aethylalcohol and found in both instances an increased motility of the spermatozoids (page 82).

BALDWIN (1920) concludes with regard to his experiments with the higher alcohols and other substances and the dividing sea urchin eggs that dividing eggs show periods of varying susceptibility and resistance when exposed to chemical substances and to various physical conditions. From such experiments it appears that, the resistance of the eggs is least at the time when they are undergoing rapid change of form.

By using chloroform fumes on unfertilised eggs of the sea urchin O. and R. HERTWIG (1887) influenced them in such a way that later, after fructification had taken place, polyspermy occurred. Egg cells are destroyed by chloroform water.

Ether and chloroform have rather a general effect on developing fish embryos, although only a small percentage of cyclopic monsters occur. Chloretone of 0.1 causes many abnormalities. The embryos are usually small (STOCKARD 1910). Chloroform fumes retard and disturb the development of fowls eggs (FÉRÉ 1893). By remaining long in chloroform fumes later development is totally suspended. Chloroform and aether are injurious to spermatozoids of the bull (KÖLLIKER 1856).

The results of the inhalation experiments with aether on fowls by PEARL (1917) correspond with those with aethyl- and methylalcohol (cf. PEARL's tables 1,5 and 14). Here also there are many divergent totals of which the mean figures have been taken and upon which conclusions have been formed.

The group of ether treated male and ether treated female consists of four matings.

mating	eggs set	infertile	% infertile	died in shell	% died in shell	hatched	% hatched	% all eggs hatched
2105	35	34	97,1	1	100,0	0,0	0,0	0,0
2106	25	4	16,0	3	14,3	18	85,7	72,0
2107	22	6	27,3	8	50,0	8	50,0	36,4
2108	21	7	31,8	3	21,4	11	78,6	52,4

FÉRÉ (1893) finds that preliminary etherisation of fowls eggs leads to a retarded development and causes deformities.

At this point the butterfly experiments by STANDFUSS, FISCHER and others may be mentioned. By the action of aether fumes on the pupae they obtained changes in the colour of the skin of the imago (cit. O. HERTWIG 1913, cf., also O. HERTWIG 1895, alimentary poly-morphism).

In a solution of 5 % glycerine the motility of the spermatozoids of the bull stops after 112 minutes immersion (GÜNTHER). In a solution of 1% dextrin the movement of spermatozoids of the dog stops in 8 minutes (GÜNTHER). Injections of a solution of glucose and of glycerine in fowls eggs causes a teratological action. (FÉRÉ 1893).

MIRTO found seven normal embryos in 18 eggs which he injected with acetone and 10 normal embryos in 18 eggs in which water is injected.

FÉRÉ (1896) injected acetone into fowls eggs and found 98 normal embryos of 156 treated eggs, i.e. 62.9 %. He found 58 normal embryos of 72 control eggs (injected with water) i.e. 80.6 %. He is of the opinion that natural breeding of modified eggs does not give reliable experimental results (contra MIRTO).

Summary. Higher alcohols according to different investigators are more injurious than aethylalcohol. Methylalcohol is likewise more injurious than aethylalcohol. In respect to the interpretation by PEARL of the results of his experiments with methylalcohol and with aether on fowls, the same objections exist as with his interpretation of his experiments with aethylalcohol. (p. 87). Chloroform fumes are injurious to the germ cells.

11. Quinine, Strychnine, Terpentine Essence, Papaine, Hydro Cyanide, Carbolic, Hydroquinone, Phenylurethane, Peptone, Creatine

Quinine acts on the egg cells of the sea urchin, as well as on other lower organisms as a strong toxic. Upon fertilisation polyspermy ensues and great pathological changes of the blastulae arise. (O. & R. HERTWIG 1887). The development of the fertilised eggs of the sea urchin is greatly disturbed by quinine solutions. There is very little impediment of the fertilisation itself. In a solution of quinine 1 : 1000 the motility of the spermatozoids of the bull stops after 30 minutes (GÜNTHER 1909). KÖLLIKER (1856) studied the influence on the spermatozoids of the bull by immersing them in a 20 % strychnine solution. The motility stopped, but returned after the addition of 1 % solution of kitchen salt. Strychnine in weak solutions also works rapidly on non-fertilised eggs of the sea urchin. The changes in the fertilisation are clearly visible. There is great polyspermy (O. and R. HERTWIG, 1887). Strychnine has only very slight toxic action on the spermatozoids of the sea urchin. The development of the fertilized eggs of the sea urchin is only slightly impaired by strychnine (O. and R. HERTWIG 1887). G. and P. HERTWIG (1913) found afterwards that strychnine does not damage the spermatozoids of the sea urchin. O.. HERTWIG (1913) made experiments with the Rana fusca by giving strychnine nitrate and obtained corresponding res ults as with chloral hydrate (page 130).

The result of some experiments were somewhat divergent.

G. and P. HERTWIG (1913) treated spermatozoids of Rana Fusca with a 0.75 % solution of strychnine nitrate and did not obtain any developed cross-breeds as a result of fertilisation with eggs of Rana esculenta (page 130).

There are observations of the injurious influence on the human being and on animals by terpentine essence vapours. In one case POTAIN reports a late abortus (cit. FÉRÉ 1893). A short treatment of fowls eggs with terpentine fumes does not impair later development. After long treatment defects and retardation of development may occur, but such are not common. In a saturated solution of terpentine oil the motility of spermatozoids of the dog stops in 13 minutes (GÜN-THER 1907).

FÉRÉ (1895) points out that there are medicines which have an injurious action when given in larger doses, and an exciting action when the doses are smaller (page 123) and he investigated to find out whether there was any eutrophic or dystrophic action on the embryo according to the dose administered to which it is subjected. He used papaine. The result of his experiments is that with solutions of 1 : 2500 and 1 : 3000 the development was distinctly more advanced in eggs having received the papaine solutions than in control eggs. The number of fertile eggs was roughly the same. If the solution of papaine is still weaker, 1 : 3500, there is hardly any difference in the rate of development with that of control eggs. If stronger solutions e.g. 1 : 100 and 1 : 200 are used not any of the eggs develop; a solution of 1 : 400 gives a small percentage of fertile eggs (4.16 %). In the solutions up to 1 : 2000 there is a smaller number of fertile eggs than with control eggs and a small number of normal embryos and a retarded development. In his investigations of substances which might produce a suractivity of the development of the embryo FÉRÉ found that cantharidine increases the variabilility and promotes the occurrence of monstra; the development is accelerated, especially when small doses are given.

A solution of 0.2% cyanide had no influence on the activity of spermatozoids of the bull a.o. (KÖLLIKER 1856).

VAN HERWERDEN (1918) placed Daphnia pulex cultures in a 0.05 % solution of potassium cyanide. There were more broods in the same period than with control material.

Of organic antiseptics of which GÜNTHER (1907) investigated the action on the spermatozoids of some mammals, he was struck by the weak action of carbolic acid and by the strength of hydro-quinine. Lysol and creoline caused strong action. KÖLLIKER (1856) had already discovered the injurious action of creosote.

VAN HERWERDEN (1919) finds great sensitivity of the egg cells of the Daphnia in the last stages of maturity, for phenylurethane. She placed Daphnia pulex cultures in n/16000 phenylurethane. More broods were formed; maturation of eggs is acelerated. In n/4000 urethane abortive young are formed. The embryos remained in the envelopment up to the last and died quickly when taken out. An occasional Daphnia developed, was placed in water and produced healthy young.

On the basis of her investigations with Daphnia and the facts known from the literature VAN HERWERDEN believes that especially the matured egg cells are very sensitive and that these would apply to the whole of the animal world.

FÉRÉ (1896) injected a 5 % peptone solution into fowls eggs and found that about as many normal embryos developed as in control material when he injected the same quantity of distilled water. When a stronger solution of 10 %, 20 % or 25 % is injected, a smaller number of normally developed embryos was obtained.

FÉRÉ (1898) injected quantities of a 1 % creatine solution and found in 8 cases that treated eggs produced more embryos and were further developed than control eggs. In one case the number of embryos was larger, but the average degree of development was less. Of the 108 eggs after 72 hours incubation, those which were injected with aqua dest. 69 % had normal development with a mean time of about 45 hours, whilst with the 108 eggs injected with creatine there

were 81.4 % normal developments with a mean time of 47 hours. Injections with xantho-creatine produced similar results. There were
76.7 % normal developments with treated eggs and 68.7 % with
untreated eggs. The average development after 72 hours incubation
is 53.5 hours with treated eggs and 45 hours with untreated.

Summary. Quinine proved in the experiments to be a strong germ
injurious agent. The experiments with strychnine with the sea urchin
and Rana did not produce such positive signs of blastophthoric action as hydras chlorali. FÉRÉ found in papaine a substance which has
an eutrophic or a dystrophic action on the embryo according to the
dose given. Carbolic acid is a weak germ poison, hydroquinone a
strong one. Phenylurethane acts very strongly on the egg cells of
Daphnia. Creatine and Xanthocreatine, in the experiments with
fowls eggs produced a larger number of embryos and also embryos
which were further advanced in their development than control
embryos.

12. Methylene Blue

Methylene blue was the first of a series of chemical substances
which O. HERTWIG (1912) used in order to determine the action
on the germ cells of Rana. On injecting methylene blue into the
lymphoid sacks of three male Rana fusca, and after fertilisation by
the egg cells of non treated females with their sperm O. HERTWIG
found in one case besides many normal embryos 15 that were defective of which 5 permanently; the larvae were small and weak, the
tail end of some was bent. In a second experiment, the male having
been treated longer, HERTWIG obtained exclusively abnormal embryos which developed into forms with Spina bifida and as Hemithe-
rium anterius ROUX respectively. Of the second testicle the spermatozoids were still treated afterwards with a methylene blue solution.
Also in this experiment all embryos differed from control material,
but the changes were not so great. The development was slower, the
larvae were not so motile; there were some Spina bifida and finally
they all developed hydrops and ascites. In this experiment it is a
question of the effect of a single action of short duration.

The results of these experiments with methylene blue correspond
greatly with similar experiments with radium and mesothorium that
this author made. The most remarkable thing in the experiments with

radium is that with strong doses injury to the germ cells is apparently slighter; from the outward appearances the larvae are normal, although small. O. HERTWIG and his collaborators (GÜNTHER HERTWIG), were able to determine that with strong doses the spermatozoids practically died out, and a parthenogenetic development took place.

MAC DOUGAL (1914) treated the embryo sacks of seedlings with methylene blue and potassium iodine (page 121) and obtained some individuals unlike the parental strain.

G and P. HERTWIG (1913) treated spermatozoids of Rana fusca with a 0.05 % solution of methylene blue and afterwards fertilised with them the eggs of Rana esculenta. Some cross products developed and reached the age of 15 days. They succumbed from ascites. This successful further development is a proof of a partial preclusion of the sperm-chromatine (page 130).

By the immersion of spermatozoids of the fish Gobius jozo in methylene blue, the course of later fecundation is disturbed; many deformities arise. Some embryos develop into normal animals. (page 145).

Treatment of spermatozoids with methylene green produced no modifications of the later fertilisation (G. and P. HERTWIG 1913). Crossing with fishes of the same family was not successful, nor with treated sperm.

In one experiment, where the spermatozoids of the sea urchin were placed in a solution of methylene blue, there were many deformities; in a second experiment development progressed practically normally.

Further in another similar experiment there were great differences. Besides embryos with serious defects in development there were always some which developed normally. O. HERTWIG also noticed this and points out that the varying influence is brought about by the chemical substances in contradistinction to the uniform influence by irradiation (cf. however GOLDSCHMIDT 1929). There is delay and irregularity of the division, formation of stereoblastulae and stereogastrulae.

G. and P. HERTWIG (1913) find that after treating the spermatozoids of the sea urchin for one hour in a 1 % solution of methylene blue, the fertilised eggs in general are uniformly disturbed in development; in cases of a long immersion the results vary; in some experiments the result is better than in the cases of short immersion. There was not a great variation of deformities, and partheno-genetical larvae were not obtained.

Spermatozoids immersed in the methylene blue for 16 to 18 hours died in great numbers. Yet in most of the experiments there are some fertilised eggs which develop and become normal embryos. There is no parthenogenesis here; the embryos are not small and do not differ from control embryos. The authors suppose that after a lengthy action of methyleneblue all spermatozoids of which the nucleus has been injured by this chemical, die. Only those spermatozoids whose nuclear structure is not susceptible to methylene blue remain alive and fertilise eggs which develop normally. By a lengthy immersion in methyleneblue there is a selection of the methylene blue "proof" spermatozoids (EHRLICH).

One fact remains unexplained and that is that when fertilising the treated spermatozoids the first division begins later than with control material. G. and P. HERTWIG take it that the methyleneblue "proof" spermatozoids have, moreover, the peculiarity of retarding the fertilisation. This is therefore a second hypothesis.

This second hypothesis is a real auxiliary hypothesis. G. and P. HERTWIG found as a result of the action of different chemical substances on the spermatozoids, that the later fertilisation proceeds slowly and that malformations occur. They consider both the phenomena as a consequence of the injurious action of the chemical substances.

The authors in their experiments with methyleneblue obtained a paradoxical result (lengthy immersion and sometimes good results, yet much retardation) and both explain the good results and the retardation by selection.

The necessity of having to accept this auxiliary hypothesis makes the whole explanation very weak. The results were moreover not general.

Summary. Methylene blue is a powerful germ injuring agent. With Rana crossing experiments were successful, which yields a proof of the highly blastophthoric action of methylene blue (just as with hydras chlorali).

In the experiments with sea urchins and fishes there is a highly retarded development and many malformations. There was great individual variability and a lack of uniformity in the results of the experiments. Ray-treatment yields a more uniform influence.

G. and P. HERTWIG also obtained varying results. Sometimes they find with long treatment great mortality and some embryos which develop normally. They take it that there are some germ cells among them which are methylene blue "proof" (EHRLICH) and that those which are susceptible die. The methylene blue resistent germ cells have, moreover, the peculiarity of retarding fertilisation.

13. Alkalis, Acids, Salts

It was shown very early that immobile spermatozoids show renewed activity by the addition of potassium or natron hydroxide and that acids on the contrary have an injurious action on the spermatozoids (QUATREFAGES 1850, KÖLLIKER 1856)).

GÜNTHER (1909) who worked much more accurately found with a $1^0/_{00}$ KOH solution an immediate stoppage of movement (GÜNTHER means by "immediate" in less than 20 seconds). With weaker solutions 1 : 2000 to 1 : 10000 the movement in two series of experiments lasted 40 seconds to $2\frac{1}{2}$ minutes and 17 minutes to 31 minutes respectively. NH_3 and $Ca(OH)_2$ have a weaker action than KOH.

When GÜNTHER added alkali (1 : 5000, KOH) to the solutions of different substances in which spermatozoids had become immobile after some time, he often found there was a temporary return of motility. With some substances, sublimate, formaldehyd this is not possible, with hydroquinone it is (page 136). The renewed activity is only temporary, it is not a restitutio ad integrim as with acids (page 141). Sublimate and formaldehyd are therefore, according to GÜNTHER, heavy sperm poisons.

TEICHMANN (1903) treated spermatozoids of sea urchins with caustic potassium solution. The damaged sperma chromatine does not fuse with the nucleus of the egg, but the latter conducts the first and sometimes the second division independently.

It is very detrimental for the development of fowls eggs to remain in ammonia fumes (FÉRÉ 1899).

In GÜNTHER's experiments with sperms of the dog, the bull and the stallion, most of the acids of a strength of $1^0/_{00}$ still act paralytically.

Acid boricum, which is known as a sperm killing agent, showed the weakest action of all acids investigated. Acetic acid, hydrochloric acid, nitric acid and sulphuric acid ($1\ ^0/_{00}$) stop the movement in about 40 minutes.

Of the acids E. ROST (1927) discusses boric acid and its action on the muscles of the uterus. Borax is known as a sal uterinum (abortificient), yet it has already been acknowledged by BINSWANGER on the basis of experiments with animals and observations with human beings to have no result.

The resistance of the spermatozoids of man to acid citricum and to hydroquinone is greater than with those of the dog (GÜNTHER 1909).

In LOEB's experiments (1896) it appeared that the egg of the fish Fundulus is very sensitive to the action of carbonic acid.

When GÜNTHER whilst experimenting with sperm of the dog which had lost its motility in a solution of $1\ ^0/_{00}$ citric acid and $0.9^0/_0$ NaCl, added 1 : 5000 KOH to the solution, making it slightly alcalic, he perceived that the movement of the spermatozoids returned and that they became just as active as control sperm. The other acids also showed the same action.

The standstill brought about to the spermatozoids by the diluted acids, is therefore only a trance which also appears with hyper and hypisotonic salt solutions.

If a little alcali is given to old sperm there is a revival of activity. This can be explained by the fact that fresh sperm is alcalic and gradually reacts acidly.

Acids strongly diluted do not destroy the spermatozoids, but only stop their movement; by adding alcali their movement is revived. Real sperm poisons are several metal salts, antiseptics and substances which possess a strong power of reduction.

GÜNTHER investigated the reaction of the sperma of the human being towards kitchen salt solutions. With a concentration of 0.9 % is the optimum of the duration of motility.

Injection of a solution of kitchen salt in fowls eggs has a teratological action. Some embryos die, others show deformities. (FÉRÉ 1893).

By immersion in a solution of kitchen salt of 0.6—1 %, the development of fertilised frogs eggs is disturbed. Development is retarded, the gastrulation is disturbed and many deformities are formed (spina bifida, anencephali, O. HERTWIG 1895).

The defects with embryos of Siredon pisciformis (Axolotl) are not so strong and are limited there to the central nervous system, so that the embryos can be bred further. LOEB interrupted the development of sea urchins eggs by placing them in a solution of kitchen salt (cit. O. HERTWIG). LOEB studied the solutions in which the fertilisation of invertebrates took place (Echinodermata) and was able by means of chemical agents to induce these lower animals to develop parthenogenetically (cf also O. HERTWIG page 137, 138).

MORGAN obtained a deviating course of the gastrulation process with frogs by placing blastulae of frogs in salt solutions of 0.3—1.0%. (cit. O. HERTWIG).

OTTO WARBURG (1910) studied the oxydation process in the fertilized and unfertilized eggcell of the sea urchin. He put the egg in an artificial salt solution and added caustic soda (NaOH); then the growth stopped, but there was a high consumption of oxygen.

Fertilized sea urchin eggs die soon, if they are put in a solution of kitchen-salt of the same strength as seawater. If one adds to the salt solution a little Ca, Zn or Pb-ions, the poisonous effect of the saltsolution is nullified (LOEB). In the same way fertilized sea urchin eggs die in a solution of kitchen salt that is isotonic with seawater, unless one adds a trace of natriumcyanide (WARBURG, 1910). According to WARBURG the poisonous effect of the kitchensalt solution is explained by the very strong increase of the oxydation process in the living cell. Small quantities of Cu-, Ag- and Au-ions paralyze in sea-water the development of fertilized seaurchin eggs. LOEB investigated in many experiments the effect of chemical substances on the development of the fertilized egg cell.

HERBST bred eggs of the sea urchin in solutions of lithioncarbonate and obtained many malformations (cit. O. HERTWIG).

STOCKARD (1909) obtained cyclopean individuals in fish which had developed in solutions containing magnesium (Mg Cl_2).

GÜNTHER (1907) traced the influence of a large number of different salts on spermatozoids. He was struck by the weak action of lead and ferro salts and the strong action of silver and mercury salts. He finds in his investigations with sperm of stallions, bulls and dogs very divergent individual resistance.

Neutral alkali salts are similar in their action on spermatozoids as kitchen salt, and are just as little injurious. They are very sensitive for the concentration. Acid and alkali reacting salt solutions are quicker in stopping the mobility than neutral ones.

Alkali salts of various aromatic acids may, also as a neutral solution, quickly paralyze the mobility of spermatozoids.

Water is also a sperm poison. KÖLLIKER (1856) already wrote long ago that by adding a few drops of water to the sperma, movement stops. The spermatozoids are apparently dead. After adding a natrium salt the spermatozoids again become active. KÖLLIKER found that the motility returns after adding many substances which favourably influence the movement of the spermatozoids, such as blood serum, sugar, albumen, ureum, glycerine, kitchen salt, potassium solution. Solution of potassium acts least in this respect.

In bovine serum the movement of spermatozoids of the dog is still to be seen after 94 minutes. In rabbit serum it stops in 5 minutes. This is a striking difference (GÜNTHER).

Summary. Weak solutions of alkali often restore the activity of spermatozoids which had stopped after a stay in acids or other chemicals. In a somewhat stronger solution ($1\ ^0/_{00}$) of potassium hydroxide the mobility stops almost immediately.

Most acids of a solution of $1\ ^0/_{00}$ work paralytically and almost immediately on spermatozoids.

With real germ poisons, sublimate, formaldehyd and other metal salts the movement of the spermatozoids does not return after the addition of alkali.

Non-isotonic solutions of kitchen salt react injuriously on the development of different lower animals; many malformations arise.

---

[1]) BLUHM (1930) gives a short report of an extensive experiment, that comprises 32300 albino mice and where special attention was given to the correspondence of experiment and control animals. Males were injected with 0.2 ccm of a 15 per cent aethylalcohol solution six times a week. The offspring received no alcohol and were watched till the 8th generation.

BLUHM finds a great prenatal mortality that appears in small litters. There is a great mortality of the young and a somewhat greater mortality of the grandchildren of the alcoholized males in the suckling age. This mortality is progressively smaller with the grand-grand-children up to and including the 7th generation. There is a small mortality of the progeny of alcoholized males at the age of 3—8 weeks. This mortality is evidently greater in the whole further life with the males and up to 3/4 of a year with the females. The body-weight is somewhat smaller up to one year with the males of treated males and up to 13 weeks with the females. There is often a general weakness. There is a great infantile mortality with the young of matings of treated males and non-treated females no matter of which generation the treated male was.

BLUHM concludes that there is in this experiment a blastophthory in the sense of mutations i.e. hereditary changes of the germplasm. It is her opinion that the male exercises the greatest influence, so the mutations are located in the sexchromosomes. This experiment will have to be judged when the full publication has appeared.

DISCUSSION AND CONCLUSIONS

The study of the literature published about different germ poisons has shown us that lead, thallium, iodine, nicotine, chloral hydrate, methylene blue etc. have a considerable injurious action as germ poisons. The germ injurious effect of alcohol (see page 76, 111) is accepted by most authors, it is doubted by some and denied by a few.

Among the germ poisons named above, thallium and methylene blue have no significance as far as the human being is concerned. In our review we have discussed further a number of poisons which have been studied experimentally which are practically also of no significance for man. It is, however, desirable when prescribing medicine for persons to think of other possible actions of it.

The germ poisoning action in the narrow sense, thus action on the germ cells before the fertilisation, is especially prominent if only the male before mating, resp. only the male gametes before fertilisation have been treated with a germ poison. Such experiments were made by the HERTWIGS with different chemical substances. COLE and BACHHUBER and WELLER used lead. BILSKI, STOCKARD and others used alcohol.

A strong germ poisonous effect on the male sexual glands was ascertained in the experiments with thallium by HECKE, with iodine by ADLER and with nicotine by HOFSTÄTTER. In all these cases far reaching anatomical modifications in the testicles of the experimental animals were found; changes which coincide with those brought about by ray treatment. Anatomical changes of the testicles in cases of chronic alcoholism of man have been specially written about by BERTHOLET and by KYRLE, SCHOPPER and WEICHSELBAUM.

O. HERTWIG as a result of his experiments with radium treatment and the action of chemical substances on spermatozoids, considers as chemical germ injury, a somewhat altered constitution of the spermatozoids i.e. of the idioplasm in a pathological direction.

It is not possible to see any changes in the spermatozoids through the microscope; however, it appears that if these spermatozoids, which remain motile and are capable of fertilisation, are brought into contact with normal eggs the process of development shows a series of disturbances (page 137).

In some cases the germ injurious action by ray treatment and also by the action of chemical substances (chloral hydrate) goes so far as to practically destroy the chromatine of the spermatozoids, and when these spermatozoids unite with eggs parthenogenetical development arises (G. and P. HERTWIG).

Disturbed development of eggs which are fertilised with spermatozoids which have been exposed to the influence of chemical substances is a clear example of blastophthory.

O. HERTWIG considers the fact that injurious action of different substances gives the same result. The reaction which follows physical or chemical stimulants is not defined by the nature of the material used but by the characters of the living matter (spermatozoids and egg cells).

HERTWIG also paid much attention to the fact that the influence of chemical substances shows great individual variation: the results of the experiments are very different. He infers that this great variable individual resistance of the spermatozoids against the action of various chemical substances is due to the varying permeability of the spermatozoid-walls.

Where EHRLICH speaks of arsenic resisting (arsenic proof) trypanosoma races and considers this resistance as an acquired immunity, O. HERTWIG suggests against this opinion the possibility that we have simply to do with individual variability, thus with an individual different resistance.

We have, when discussing the germ injurious action of alcohol, also accepted the possibility that there is a variable resistance of the germ cells and that some of these cells are not injured and may be called alcohol "proof" (page 110).

G. and P. HERTWIG in respect to the action of methylene blue accept a selective agency.

FÉRÉ, who studied the action of many chemical substances on the development of the fertilized eggs brooded afterwards, is of the opinion that some substances in small doses may have a favourable action. He distinguishes an entrophic and a dystrophic action (Féré, (Féré, p. 119). This is found with terpentine essence and with papaine. Furthermore there is great individual variability. He found the deleterious action of nicotine very great, yet some embryos developed well. In the case of creatine he found mostly that a large number of embryos developed and that development was far advanced. Creatine would therefore in particular have an exciting action. For nicotine we must take it that it has a paralysing effect and an exciting action when given in weak solutions and for some resistant germ cells.

STIEVE mentions an all-or-nothing rule with respect to the results of his caffein experiments.

These are the same phenomena as are met with in the action of alcohol (page 87) and we repeat that it seems to us not correct to speak of selective action here. Selection has not actually been established anywhere. JOHANNSEN (1926, page 670) writing about heredity by adaptation, which expression is used in a somewhat different meaning than with selection, states that the conclusion in many cases of adaptation to environment is insufficiently motived, it is even an unproved opinion. JOHANSSEN cites WENT who showed with certain water plants which live in an abundance of water that the solid manner of cleavage cannot be gradually created here.

The discussion on adaptation and selection by WILLIAM BATESON in the introduction of his renowned book Materials for the Study of Variation (1894, p. 10—13) is also very important. „It is most important that its proper use and scope should be understood", BATESON says. And „There is need for great reserve" „in dealing with questions of adaptation more than usual caution is needed". „ . . . . Since at the present time the conclusions arrived at in this field are being allowed to pass unchallenged to a place among the traditional beliefs of science, it is well to remember that the evidence for these beliefs is far from being of the nature of a proof." „We live not only by virtue of, but also in spite of what we are"... We can only get an indefinite knowledge of adaptation, which for the purposes of our problem (the test of the theory of natural selection) is not an advance beyond the original knowledge that organisms are all more or less adapted to their circumstances".

PEARL has dealt quite recently with this question. He writes (1930, p, 181): "No proof of the effectiveness of natural selection in altering a race can be logically complete until it has been demonstrated that there are genetic differences between survivors and eliminated, as well as somatic differences". (see also PEARL, p. 184).

I therefore think, taking this into consideration, that it is better not to speak of selection in respect to the effect of alcohol.

In the experiments with PEARL's fowls, the results of which are contestable (page 87), it is found when crossing treated males with treated females that a small number of chickens are born and that these are in good condition. Selection could be spoken of, if it transpired that also these chickens should have a strong resistance against alcohol when they were full grown and that their offspring would not be influenced or only little by alcohol.

The experiments of PEARL correspond with those of HARRISON, DANFORTH, HERTWIG, FÉRÉ, BLUHM a.o. for so far these investigators also found in their experiments germ cells which had a strong resisting power against the action of the different chemical substances used by them.

It is therefore also necessary not to draw any far reaching conclusion from the results of these experiments, because the results thereof are so variable. Especially with the experiments with fowls very divergent results were obtained; also with non-treated material the number of fertilised eggs of chickens that died in the shell and of chickens that hatched, is sometimes very different.

The experiments which have most certainly shown the existence of resistant races are according to my opinion those made by HANSON and HEYS. HANSON commenced with 6 female white rats (albino rats). Of these alcohol treated female rats five were sterile or did not produce any viable offspring (page 99), the sixth female proved to be a slightly better breeder than control material and produced the whole alcohol line. In 10 generations HANSON and HEYS exposed this line to alcoholic fumes; after 10 generations the changes in respect to the control material were zero or minimal. It is possible that it concerns a very resistant race.

It is somewhat premature to conclude a selective action of alcohol. There are some cells which are resistant to germ poisons and which probably do not become injured, yet there are many which suffer some harm, which injury leads to the occurrence of abortions, still births, and degenerate newly born offspring which remain inferior in their later life. That this group disappears through selective action, is not shown. It is therefore much better to speak of individual variability and varying resistance. This does not presume anything.

The fact that defects are always present in the human population, whereas if their existence only rested on heredity, they according to their little chance of mating, would die out, pleads for the significance of general working injuries, such as alcoholism of the parents (WEINBERG p. 33). There is more reason with regard to alcohol and the other germ poisons to speak of degeneration of the progeny than of selection.

The individual variability of the test animals and of the germ cells has been experienced by many investigators. To those already mentioned we add JORÈS, who found it with lead and also OLIVER; HECKE found it with thallium, ADLER with iodine and VAN HERWERDEN with urethane.

There are still some important points which can be touched upon. Different investigators state that there is quick recovery in respect to successive generations, if the use of the poison is discontinued. This was reported by WELLER in connection with the use of lead; O. and R. HERTWIG found the same with nicotine and hydras chlorali and BILSKI with alcohol.

There is little known of the injury to offspring in later life by the different germ poisons, and it is very difficult to determine. WELLER reports that in his experiments with lead with guinea pigs, the surviving young are permanently inferior.

The knowledge of all the other germ poisons does not throw much light on the knowledge of parental alcoholism. Lead is a strong germ poison which is proved by the number of abortions and stillbirths.

The deviations which have been observed up to the present with offspring of parents injured by germ poisons and which offspring are suitable for propagation are all only phaenotypical. Changes of the genotype, thus of the hereditary factors, have not been determined. (For ray treatment see H. J. MÜLLER 1928, for treatment with high temperatures R. GOLDSCHMIDT, 1929).

Our knowledge of the action of the germ poisons is very incomplete. that of alcohol is uncertain in its range owing to the divergent results of different investigators. Further investigations are necessary and form an attractive task for scientific researchers. The method, especially owing to the increase of our knowledge of heredity, has been considerably improved.

Tracing the causes of illnesses is a high task of scientific investigation. This is the way which leads to pathogenesis and prophylaxis. (VON KRAFFT EBING).

———

LITERATURE

A. Alcohol

1930. ALKOHOL u. VERERBUNG. Bericht üb. die von der D. Reichshauptstelle gegend. Alkoholismus am 19. Okt. 1929 usw. Berlin Neuland-Verlag 31 S. (cit. Polisch).

1925. ALLEN cf. PEARL.

1911. R. ALLERS. Noch einmal die Frage der Trinkerkinder, u.s.w. Archiv f. Rass. u. Ges. Biol. S. 268 u. 655. Bd. 8.

1913. ALLERS. Ueb. die directe Alcohol-Erblichkeit. Arch. f. Rass. Ges. Biol. X, 263.

1918. K. AMADIAN cf. PREISIG.

1901. ANTON. Alkoholismus und Erblichkeit. Bericht über das 8. internat. Kongress gegen den Alkoholismus, Wien. April 1901. S. 105.

1902. G. ARCHDALL REID. Alcoholism a study in heredity. London. BALlière a. o. (cit. AMADIAN and PREISIG).

1912. G. ARCHDALL REID. Recent Researches on Alcoholism. BEDROCK. (cit. AMADIAN and PREISIG).

1917. ADA H. ARLITT and H. G. WELLS. The effect of the alcohol on the reproductive tissues. The journal of experimental med. Vol. 26, p. 769.

1899. R. ARRIVÉE. Influence de l'alcoolisme sur la dépopulation. THÈSE, Paris.

1878. BAER. Der Alkoholismus. Berlin, 1878, p. 268.

1910. BAYERTHAL. Zur Aetiologie des angeborenen Schwachsinns. Neur. Cent. 29. Jhrg., S. 1023.

1909. E. BERTHOLET. De l'influence de l'alcoolisme chronique sur le testicule humain. Proc. 12. intern. Congress on Alcoholism, London, p. 294.

1909. E. BERTHOLET. Ueber Atrophie des Hodens bei chronischem Alkoholismus. Centralbl. f. allg. Path. u. path. Anat., Bd. 20, S. 1062.

1921. E. BERTHOLET. Alterations anatomo-pathologiques observées á l'autopsie de 100 alcooliques chroniques. Bericht über das XIII. intern. Kongress gegen den Alkohol, Haag.

1901. BEZZOLA. Statistische Untersuchingen über die Rolle des Alkohols bei der Entstehung des originären Schwachsinns. Bericht über das 8. intern. Kongress. gegen den Alkoholismus, Wien. April, 1901. S. 109.

1911. BIANCHI (STÜBER).

1921. F. BILSKI. Ueber Blastophthorie durch Alkohol. Mit Versuchen am Frosch. Arch. f. Entw. mech. Bd. 47, S. 627.

1926. F. BILSKI. Weitere Untersuchungen über den Einfluss der Alkoholisierung der Eltern auf die Nachkommenschaft beim Frosch. Archiv f. Entw. mech. 108. Bd. S. 680.

1899. O. BINSWANGER. Die Epilepsie. In NOTHNAGEL's Handb. XII, I, 1. Wien.

1904. O. BINSWANGER und E. SIEMERLING. Lehrbuch. der Psychiatrie. G. FISCHER, Jena.

1922. O. BINSWANGER. Die Pathogenese und Prognose der Epilepsie. München und Wien. Nr. 39 u. 40.

1908. AGN. BLUHM. Familiärer Alkoholismus und Stillfähigkeit. Archiv f. Rass. u. Ges. biol. 5. Jhrg., S. 635.

1921. AGN. BLUHM. Ueber einen Fall experimenteller Verschiebung des Geschlechtsverhältnisses bei Säugetieren. Sitz. ber. Pr. Akad. d. Wiss. Jhrg. 1921, II, S. 549. (also 1924, Arch. f. R. u. G. Bi. 16, 1).

1922. AGN. BLUHM. Alkohol und Nachkommenschaft. Sammelber. Z. f. ind. Vererb. u. Abst. 1. Bd. 28, S. 75 (ook in „Die Alkoholfrage" 18. Jhrg. S. 12, 1922).

1928. AGN. BLUHM. Diskussion z. Vortr. MAC DOWELL. Verh. 5. Intern. Kongress f. Vererb. wiss. Berlin 1927, Bd. II, S. 1086.

1930. A. BLUHM. Ueber exogene Keimschädigungen. Münch. med. W. N. 37, p. 1596. (Also Arch. f. Rass. Ges. Bi. 34 and J. F. Lehmann, München).

1913. G. C. BOLTEN. Pathogenese und Therapie der Epilepsie. Mon. f. Psych. u. Neurol. Bd. 33, S. 119.

BONHOEFFER. Klinische und anatomische Beitragen zur Kenntn. der Alkohol delirien. Mon. schr. Psych. u. Neur. I.

1929. M. BOSS. Z. Frage der erbbiol. Bedeutung des Alkohols. Mon.schr. Psychiatr. u. Neur. 72, 264.

1912. CH. BOUCHARD et G. H. ROGER. Nouv. Traité de Pathologie générale. Tome I et II, Paris.

1900. BONIN et GARNIER. Altérations du tube séminifère au cours de l'alcoolisme expérimental chez le rat blanc. C. R. Soc. biol. Paris. p. 23.

1921. BOULENGER. La criminalité et l'alcoolisme d'un des parents. Verh. int. Kongr. g. d. Alc. Lausanne.

1928. K. H. BOUMAN, see VERWEY.

1885. BOURNÉVILLE et SÉGLAS. Des Familles d'idiots. Arch. de neurol. T. 10, p. 186 et 347.

1900. BOURNÉVILLE. Comptes rendus du service des enfants idiots, épileptiques et arriérés de Bicêtre pendant l'année 1899.

1910. BOURNÉVILLE. Recherches clin. et thérap. sur l'épilepsie, l'hystérie et l'idiotie. Paris.

1918. W. BOVEN. Religiosité et épilepsie. Schweiz. Arch. f. Neur. u. Psych. IV, p. 153.

1899. BRATZ. Alkohol und Epilepsie. Allg. Zeitschr. f. Psychiatrie, Bd. 56, S. 334.

1901. BRATZ und HEBOLD. Deutsche med. Wochenschr. 1901, Nr. 36.

1908. BRATZ. Zur Aetiologie der Epilepsie. Neur. Cent., S. 1063.

1903. H. BREYER. Ueber die Einwirkung verschiedener einatomiger Alkohole auf das Flimmerepithel und die motorische Nervenfaser. PFLÜGER, Arch. 99, S. 481.

1928. C. BRUGGER. Die erbbiologische Stellung der Pfropfschizophrénie. Zeitschr. f. d. ges. Neur. und Psych., 113, 348.

1924. O. BUMKE. Lehrbuch der Geisteskrankheiten. Allg. Teil. 1. Bd., S. 279. O. BUMKE. Die exogenen Vergiftungen des Nervensystems. LEWANDOWSKY, Handb. d. Neur. III.

1904. G. VON BUNGE. Alkoholismus und Degeneration. VIRCHOW's Archiv, Bd. 175, S. 185.

1904. G. VON BUNGE. Alkoholvergiftung und Degeneration. Ein Vortrag, Leipzig.

1908. G. VON BUNGE. Bemerkungen u.s.w. Arch. f. Rass. u. Ges. biol. 5. Jhrg., S. 656.

1909. G. VON BUNGE. Die zunehmende Unfähigkeit der Frauen ihre Kinder zu stillen. Ein Vortrag 6. aufl. München.

1904/5. CARLO CENI. Influenza dell' alcoolismo sul potere di procreare e sui descendenti. Riv. sperim. di Freniatria, 30, 339 (cit. NICE) Prof. Neur. Cent. p. 566.

1873. CHARPENTIER. Influence de l'alcool de la nourrice sur les convulsions du nourrisson. Bull. de la Soc. protect. de l'enfant, 1873.

1914. L. J. COLE and C. L. DAVIS. The effect of alcohol on the male germ cells etc. Science, N.S., 39, p. 476.

1913. A. COLLINS. The hereditary transmission of epilepsy. Epilepsia. Vol. 4, p. 365.

1919. C. H. DANFORTH. Evidence of germ cell selection. Journ. of exper. Zool. Vol. 28, p. 385.

1925. C. H. DANFORTH. Alcohol and the sex ratio in mice, p. 305. Proc. Soc. Exp. Biol. med. 23, 1925, 1926.

1911. CH. DAVENPORT and D. F. WEEKS. A first study of inheritance of epilepsy. The journal of nerv. and ment. disease, Vol. 38, p. 641.

1886. J. DÉJERINE. L'Hérédité dans les maladies du système nerveux, Paris.

1890. R. DEMME. Ueber den Einfluss des Alkohols auf den Organ. des Kindes. Rede, Stuttgart, 1891.

1899. J. DEMOOR. Les enfants anormaux et la criminologie. Rev. d. l'Univ. de Bruxelles, Avril 1899. (cit. FÉRÉ).

1929. DERVIEUX, SZUMLANSKI et DESVILLE, H. Méthode pour la recherche tardive, du degrée d'intoxication alcool. de la nourrice. Soc. méd. lég. France. Ann. de med. leg. 1929, 7, p. 501.

1905. O. DIEM. Die psychoneurotische erbliche Belastung der Geistesgesunden und der Geisteskranken. Arch. f. Rass. u. Ges. Biol. II, S. 215 u. 336.

1920. R. Dittler. Studien z. Physiologie der Befruchtung. I. Die Sterilisierung des weibl. Tierkörpers durch parenterale Spermazufuhr. Z.f. Biol. 72, 273.

1928. Rud. Dreikurs. Wien. Die Entwicklung der psychischen Hygiene in Wien. Unter besonderer Berücksichtigung der Alkoholiker und Psychopathen. (Selbstmörder-) fürsorge. Allgem. Zeitschr. f. Psychiatrie u. psych. gerichtl. Medizin, 88. Bd. S. 469.

1910. R. L. Dugdale. The Jukes. A study in Crime, Pauperism, Disease and Heredity, (1875) 4. ed. G. P. Putman's Sons, New-York, London.

1880. Matth. Duncan. Transact. Edinb. Obst. Soc., p. 105 (cit. Van der Hoeven).

1912. Duval et Mulon. Pathogénie générale de l'embryon. Tératogénie. In Bouchard et Roger. 2 vol.

1880. M. G. Echeverria. Marriage and Hereditariness of Epileptics. Journal of ment. science. Vol. 26, p. 346.

1881. M. G. Echeverria. Alcoholic Epilepsy. Journ. of ment. science. Vol. 26, p. 489.

1909. E. M. Elderton.The relative strength of nurture and nature.Eugenics Labor. Lect. Ser. III, London.

1915. W. Eliassow. Erbliche Belastung und Entwicklung von Hilfsschulkindern in Königsberg. Arch. f. Psych. u. Nervenkrankh. Bd. 56, S. 123.

1928. J. L. Entres. Vererbung. Keimschädigung. Im Handb. d. Geisteskrankheiten. Herausgeg. v. O. Rumke, 1. Bd. Allg. Teil, I, S. 279 (Lit.)

1838. E. Esquirol. Des maladies mentales. T. II, p. 72, Paris.

1914. A. W. Fairbanks. A Study of the Etiology in One Hundred and Seventy-Five Children. Boston med. and surg. Journ. 170, p. 521.

1884. Ch. Féré. La famille névropathique. Arch. de neur. T. 7, p. 1 en 173.

1890. Ch. Féré. Les épilepsies et les épileptiques. Paris

1893. Ch. Féré. Note sur la fréquence et sur la distribution de quelques difformités de la peau chez les épileptiques. C. r. soc. biol. Paris, p. 57 (naevi pigmentaires et saillants, n. vascul. taches pigm.).

1894. Ch. Féré. Poulets vivants provenant d'oeufs ayant subi des injections d'alcool éthylique dans l'albumen. Comptes rendus de la soc. biol. Paris, p. 646.

1910. M. Ferrari. Histologische Untersuch. am Zentr. nerv. syst. von Abkömmlingen chron. alkohol. Tiere. Mon. schr. f. Psych. u. Neur., Bd. 28, S. 483.

1929. Fetscher. Vererbung u. Alkohol. Int. z. Alk. H. 6, p. 3.

1930. M. Fischer, Der Alkoholmissbruach. Das kommende Geschlecht. Bd. 4, H. 3.

1911. A. Forel. Alkohol und Keimverderbnis, S. 162. Bericht über das XIII. Kongress gegen dem Alkoholismus, im Haag, S. 162.

1911. A. Forel. Alkohol und Keimzellen (Blastophthorische Entartung). München. med. Wochenschr. II, 2596. (Vortr. Kongr. geg. d. Alk., im Haag).

1924. G. P. FRETS. Alcohol en Kiembeschadiging. Voordracht. De Wegwijzer.

1925. G. P. FRETS. Over ontaarding. Ned. Tijdschr. voor Geneesk. 69e jrg. I, blz. 1699.

1926. G. P. FRETS. Alcohol en erfelijkheid. Mensch en Maatschappij. 1926.

1927. G. P. FRETS. Alcohol en eugeniek. Feestbundel dr. H. KLINKERT. Brusse, Rotterdam.

1928. G. P. FRETS. Alcohol. Individu en Gemeenschap.

1929. G. P. FRETS. Erfelijkheidsonderzoek van vijf gevallen van de ziekte van VON RECKLINGHAUSEN. Genetica, p. 347.

1931. G. P. FRETS. Kiemvergiften. Mensch en Maatschappij. (also Keim-gifte. Ploetz-Festschrift, Arch. f. Rass. Ges. Biol. 34, 1930).

1907. GADELIUS. Alkohol und Geisteskrankheit. Anti-Alcohol-Congres, Stockholm.

1927. R. GANTER. Ueber Erblichkeit bei der Epilepsie und dem Schwach-sinn. Arch. f. Psych. Bd. 81, S. 395.

1925. R. GAUPP. Die Unfruchtbarmachung geistig und sittlich Kranker und Minderwertiger.

1907. GEELVINK. Ueber die Grundlagen der Trunksucht. Neurol. Centralbl. S. 351.

1912. PAUL LE GENDRE. Hérédité. M. BOUCHARD & ROGER. 2 vol.

1928. K. GERUM. Beitrag zur Frage der Erbbiologie der genuïnen Epilepsie, der epileptoiden Erkrankungen und der epileptoïden Psychopathic. Zeitschr. f. d. ges. Neur. u. Psych. Bd. 115, S. 319.

1910. H. GODDARD. Heredity of feeble-mindedness. American Breeder's Magaz. Vol. 1, p. 165, N. 3. Washington. (*ref. E. Rüd.* Arc. f. R. G. B. 1911).

1912. H. B. GODDARD. Die Familie Kallikak. Eine Studie über die Ver-erbung des Schwachsinns. Berecht. d. Uebers. v. K. WILKER, 1914. Beitr. z. Kinderforsch. u. Erz. Beitr. z. Z. f. Kinderforsch. H. 116.

1896. K. GRASSMANN. Kritischer Überblick über die gegenw. Lehre von der Erblichkeit der Psychosen. Allg. Zeitschr. f. Psychiatrie. Bd. 52, S. 960.

1923. C. GRAVE. Cf. HANSON and HANDY.

1899. N. GRÉHANT. Recherches expérimentales sur l'intoxication par l'alcool éthylique. Comptes rendus soc. biol., Paris p. 808.

1900. N. GRÉHANT. Recherches expérim. sur l'alcool aigu. Journ. anat. physiol. 36, 150.

1887. GRENIER. La descendance des alcooliques. THÈSE, Paris, 1887. (cit. E. MÜLLER).

1911. W. GRUHLE. Ueber die Fortschritte in der Erkenntnis der Epilepsie in den letzten 10 Jahren. Zeitschr. f. d. ges. Neur. u. Psych. Ref. Bd. 2, S. 1.

1924. W. GRUHLE. Ueber die Fortschritte in der Erkenntnis der Epilepsie in den Jahren 1910—1920 und über das Wesen dieser Krankheit. Zeitschr. f. d. ges. Neur. u. Psych. Bd. 34, S. 1.

1926. I. GUSCHMER. Zum Problem der Erbprognosebestimmung (Epilepsie). Z. f. d. ges. Neur. u. Psych. Bd. 106, S. 258.

1929. I. Guttmann. Beitrag zur Epilepsiestatistiek Zeitschr. f. d. ges. Neur u. Psych. Bd. 118, S. 500.

1927. W. Handwerk. Der Blutalkohol nach Genuss alkoholischer Getränke unter verschiedenen Resorptionsbedingungen. Pharmak. Beitr. z. Alkoholfrage. II, 2, Jena.

1923. F. B. Hanson. Modifications in the Albino-Rat following treatment with alcohol fumes and x-rays. Proc. Am. Phil. Soc. Vol. 62, p. 301.

1923. Hanson and Handy. The Effects of Alcohol Fumes on the Albino-Rat. Amer. Nat. Vol. 57, p. 532.

1924. F. B. Hanson and F. Heys. Correlations of Body Weight, Body Length and Tail.Length in normal and alcoholic Albino-Rats. Genetics. Vol. 9, p. 368.

1925. F. B. Hanson and F. Heys. Alcohol and the sex ratio. Genetics X, p. 351.

1927. F. B. Hanson and F. Heys. Do albino-rats having ten generations of alcoholic ancestry inherit resistance to alcohol fumes? Amer. Nat. Vol. 61, p. 43.

1928. F. B. Hanson and F. Heys. Alcohol and white rats. Verh. 5. Int. Kongress. für Vererb. wissenschaft, Berlin 1927, II, S. 813.

1928. Hanson, Sholes and Heys. Alcohol and body-weight in the albino-rat. Genetics 13, 121.

1930. J. B. Hanson and Z. K. Cooper. The effects of ten generations of alcoholic ancestry upon learning ability in the albino rat. J. exp. Zool. 56, 369.

1914. F. Hartmann u. H. di Gaspero. Die Epilepsie. Handb. d. Neurologie v. Lewandowsky, 5. Bd., S. 832.

1905. J. Hartmann. Ueb. die heredit. Verhalt. b. Verbr. Mon. f. Krimin. psych. u. Strafr. ref. Bd. I. S. 493.

1929. M. Hartmann. Fortpflanzung und Befruchtung als Grundlage der Vererbung. Handbuch der Vererbungswissensch. Liefr. 6 (I A) Bd. I.

1917. A. Hauptmann. Ueber Epilepsie im Lichte der Kriegserfahrungen. Z. f. d. ges. Neur. und Psych., Bd. 36, S. 181.

1901. Hebold und Bratz. Die Rolle der Autoïntoxikation in der Epilepsie. Deutsche med. Wochenschr. Nr. 36, S. 601.

1912. Heilig und Steiner. Zur Kenntnis der Entstehungsbedingungen der genuïnen Epilepsie. Z. f. d. ges. Neur. und Psych., Bd. 9, S. 633.

1925. D. Herderschee. De oorzaken der zwakzinnigheid. Tijdschr. v. Buitengew. Onderw. Vol. 6, p. 141.

1912. D. Heron. The Feeble-minded Inebriate. The Lancet, p. 887 (a study of extreme alcoolism).

1929. M. A. van Herwerden. Erfelijkheid bij den Mensch en Eugenetiek. 2e druk, Amsterdam.

1919. G. Herxheimer. Schmaus' Grundriss d. pathol. Anatomie, 13. u. 14. Aufl., Wiesbaden.

1919. J. W. Heslop Harrison. A preliminary study of the effects of administering ethylalcohol to the Lepidopterous Insect Selenia Cilunaria with particular reference to the offspring. Journ. of Genetics. Vol. 9, p. 39, 1920.

1906. G. HEYMANS und E. WIERSMA. Beitr. z. spez. Psychologie auf Grund einer Massenuntersuchung. Zeitschr. f. Psych. 1906, Bd. 42, S. 87—127 en 258—301, spec. 259—260. Bd. 49, S. 444; Bd. 43, S. 321; Bd. 45, S. 1; Bd. 46, S. 321.

1911. H. HIGIER. Zur Pathologie der angeborenen, familiären und heredit-ären Krankheiten. Arch. f. Psychiatrie, Bd. 48, S. 41.

1903. C. F. HODGE. The influence of alcohol on growth and development. Physiol. asp. of the liq. probl. 1. Ed. J. S. BILLINGS HOIGHTON, MIF-FLIN., New-York, p. 359. (cit. NICE).

1919. P. C. T. VAN DER HOEVEN. Ziekteoorzaken in het leven voor de ge-boorte. Rede Dies, Leiden.

1909. H. HOPPE. Die Zeugung im Rausche. Zent. f. Nerv. u. Psych. 32. Jhrg., p. 161.

1912. H HOPPE. Die Tatsachen über den Alkohol. 554 S. 4. Aufl. München.

1917. R. HOUWINK HZN. De werking van alcohol op het nageslacht bij kip-pen. N. T. v. Gen. 61 jrg. I B, p. 1685.

1925. A. HUTTER. Het constitutioneel familiebeeld bij de schizophrenic. Diss. Groningen.

1901. F. IMBAULT. Contributions á l'étude de la fréquence de la tuberculose chez les alcoholiques. Thèse de Paris.

1913. J. IVANOW. Action de l'alcool sur les spermatozoïdes de mammifères. C. r. hebdomadaire et mém. d. 1. soc. de la biol. Ann. 1913, T. Ier, p. 480—482.

1910. R.VON JAKSCH. Die Vergiftungen. In NOTHNAGEL's Handbuch, 2e Aufl.

1926. G. JELGERSMA. Leerboek der psychiatrie. I, 426, 352; III, 477, 548.

1911. S. E. JELLIFFE. The hereditary and constitutional features of the dem-entia praecox make up. The Journ. of new and ment. dis. Vol. 38, p. 5.

1911. E. JENDRASSIK. Die hereditären Krankheiten. v. LEWANDOWSKY's Handbuch der Neurologie, 2. Bd., S. 321.

1914. P. JÖDICKE. Ueber die aetiol. Verhältn., Lebensdauer, allgem. Sterb-lichkeit u.s.w. bei Epileptikern. Zeitschr. f. d. Erforsch. u. Behandl. d. jugendl. Schwachs. 7, 201.

1905. JÖRGER. Die Familie Zero. Arch. f. Rass. u. Ges. Biol., 2. Jhrg., S. 494.

1918. JÖRGER. Die Familie Markus. Z. f. d. g. N. Ps. 43, 76.

1929. O. KANKELEIT. Die Unfruchtbarmachung aus rassenhygienischen und sozialen Gründen. LEHMANN's Verlag, München.

1922. KAUFMANN. Lehrbuch der Pathologie und Anatomie.

1910. W. KERN. Ueber den Einfluss des Alkohols auf die Tuberkulose; ex-perim. Untersuch. am Meerschweinchen. Zeitschr. f. Hyg. u. Infect. krankh., 66. Bd., S. 455.

1924. H. D. KING. Litter production and the sex ratio in various strains of rats. Anat. Record. Vol. 27, p. 337.

1927. H. KIONKA, Jena. Pharmakologische Beiträge z. Alkoholfrage. G. FISCHER, Jena. 1927. H. 1. Der Alkoholgehalt des menschlichen Blutes.

1903—1906. R. KOBERT. Lehrbuch der Intoxikationen. II, Stuttgart, Bd. I, 1903, Bd. II 1906, 2. Aufl.

1923. M. KOCHMANN. Alkohol. Hefter I, S. 262 (niets).

1895. J. KOLLER. Beitr. z. Erblichkeitsstatistiek der Geisteskranken im Canton Zürich, u.s.w., Arch. f. Psych., 27, S. 268.

1914. A. KOLLER. Statistisches über das Irrenwesen in der Schweiz. Z. f. d. ges. Neur. u. Psych. 26. Bd., S. 113.

1922. KOSTITSCH, A. Action de l'alcool sur les cellules séminales. Int. Zeitschr. g. d. Alkoh. 1922, P. 2. Also C. r. Soc. biol. Paris 84, 674, 1921.

1923. E. KRAEPELIN u. A. Die Wirkungen der Alkoholknappheit während des Weltkrieges. Herausgeg. v. d. Deutschen Forschungsanstalt f. Psych in München. J. SPRINGER, Berlin.

1927. E. KRAEPELIN u. JOH. LANGE. Psychiatrie. Bd. I. J. LANGE: Allg. Psych. S. 128.

1890. VON KRAFFT EBING. Psychiatrie.

1929. V. KRASUSKY. Ueber die Einwirkung des Alkoholismus auf die Kriminalität. Ref. Zent. f. d, ges. N. u. Ps. 54, 716.

1924. H. M. KROON. De erfelijkheid van drankzucht in de familie X. Ned. Tijdschr. voor Geneesk. 1e Deel, 1855; ook: Ned. Gen. Ver. Ber. No. 14, 1923.

1929. F. KÜENZI. Ueber das Wiederauftreten von Epilepsie unter den Nachkommen von Epileptikern. Monatschr. f. Psych. u. Neur. 72, 245.

1929. KÜENZI. Ueber das Wiederauftreten von Epilepsie unter den Nachkommen von Epileptikern. Mon.schr. Psychiatr. u. Neur. 72, 245.

1927. W. KÜFFNER. Epilepsie und Alkohol. Z. f. d. ges. Neur. u. Psych., Bd. 111, S. 145.

1929. KUFUSHIRO, K. Pathological changes of ovary due to lead poisoning. Trans. Japan. path. Soc. Tokyo. 19, 109. (cit. cent.Bl. path. 1930).

1930. KÜNZLER. Resultate der Trinkerheilstätte an der Thur. Allg. Zeitschr. f. Psychiatr. 92, 146.

1914. J. KYRLE und K. J. SCHOPPER. Untersuchungen über den Einfluss des Alkohols auf Leber und Hoden des Kaninchens. VIRCHOW's Archiv, Vol. 215, p. 309.

1901. P. LADRAGUE. Alcoolisme et enfants. Thèse. Fac. de méd. de Paris.

1900. F. LAITINEN. Ueber den Einfluss des Alkohols auf die Empfindlichkeit des Tier körpers für Infektionsstoff. Zeitschr. für Hyg. 24, Bd., p. 206.

1908. F. LAITINEN. Ueber die Einwirkung der kleinsten Alkoholmengen auf die Wiederständsfähigkeit des tier. Organismus mit bes. Berücksichtigung der Nachkommenschaft. Zeitschr. f. Hyg. Bd. 58, S. 139 u. 159. (Ook Congres tegen alcohol, Stockholm 1907, App., p. 81).

1909. F. LAITINEN. A. contribution to the study of the influence of alcohol on the degeneration of human offspring, p. 263. Verslag van het XIIIe Congres tegen het alcoholisme, Londen.

1926. F. LAITINEN. Der 18. Int. Kongress zur Bekämpfung des Alkoholismus in Dorpat vom 22—29 Juli 1926. Ref. Dr. K. BORNSTEIN, Berlin. Zeitschr. für ärztl. Fortbildung 1926, Nr. 22, S. 740, 2.

1879. LANCERAUX. De l'influence de l'alcoolisme des parents sur la santé des enfants. Epilepsie d'origine alcoolique. Gaz. des Hopit. 52, N. 48, p. 377.

1927. LANGE, cf KRAEPELIN.

1889. LEGRAIN. Hérédité et alcoolisme. Paris.

1895. LEGRAIN. Dégénérescence soc. et alcoolisme. Paris.

1903. LEGRAIN. Alkoholismus und Tuberkulose. Bericht über d. 9. int. Klongress gegen den Alkoholismus, Bremen, Apr. 1903, S. 55.

1922. F. LENZ. Die Neuerstehung krankhafter Anlagen. In BAUR, FISCHER, LENZ. Vol. I, p. 304.

1922. F. LENZ. Menschliche Auslese und Rassenhygiene. In BAUR, FISCHER, LENZ. Grundr. menschl. Erbl.l. u. Rass.hyg. München, Vol. 2, p. 46.

1929. A. LOKAY. Ueber die hereditären Beziehungen der Imbezillität. Z. f. d. ges. Neur. u. Psych. 122, 90.

1928. O. LÖWENSTEIN. Das psychiatrisch -erbbiologische Archiv in Bonn. Arch. f Psych. 85, 271.

1913. H. LUNDBORG. Mediz. biol. Familienuntersuchungen innerhalb eines 2232 Köpf. Bauerngeschlechts in Schweden. G. FISCHER, Jena.

1921. E. C. MAC DOWELL. The influence of alcohol on the fertility of white rats. Genetics, Vol. 7, p. 117.

1921. E. C. MAC DOWELL. Alcoholism and the growth of white rats. Genetics VII, 1922, p. 427.

1921. E. C. MAC DOWELL and E. M. VICARI. Alcoholism and the behaviour of white rats. 1. The influence of alcohlic grandparents upon mazebehaviour. Journ. exper. Zool. 33, 209.

1923. E. C. MAC DOWELL. Alcoholism and the behaviour of white rats. II. The maze behaviour of treated rats and their offspring. Journ. of exper. Zoöl., Vol. 37, p. 417 (Ook I, Vol. 33, 1921).

1924. E. C. MAC DOWELL. A method of determining the prenatal mortality in a given pregnancy of a mouse without affecting its subsequent reproduction. The anatomical Record, Vol. 27, p. 329.

1925. E. C. MAC DOWELL and E. M. LORD. The sex ratio in litters of mice classified by the total amount of prenatal mortality .Proc. Soc. f. exp. biol. a. med., New-York, p. 389.

1925. E. C. MAC DOWELL, CARLETON and E. M. LORD. Proc. Soc. exp. biol. a. med. 22, 389.

1926. E. C. MAC DOWELL and E. M. LORD. The relative viability of male and female mouse embryos. The Amer. Journ. of anat. Vol. 37, p. 127.

1926. E. C. MAC DOWELL, E. M. LORD and C. G. MAC DOWELL. The sex ratio of mice from alcoholized fathers. Proc. Soc. Exp. Biol. a. Med. Vol. 23, 1925—1926,p. 517.

1927. E. C. MAC DOWELL and E. M. LORD. Reproduction in alcoholic mice. I. Treated females. A study of the influence of alcohol on ovarian activity, prenatal mortality and sex ratio. ROUX' Archiv, 109 (4) p. 549—583.

1928. E. C. MAC DOWELL. Alcohol and Sex Ratio in Mice. Verh. 5. Int. Kongress für Vererb. wissensch., Berlin, 1927. II. S. 1081.

1880. MAGNAN. De la coëxistence de plusieurs délires de nature différente chez le même aliéné. Arch. de neur. T. 1, p. 49.

1888. A. MAIRET et COMBEMALE. Influence dégénrative de l'alcool sur la descendance. Rech. expér. Comptes rendus d. s. acad. d. sciences. T. 106, p. 667.

1926. MALEIKA. Alkohol in Königsberg. Arch. f. Psych., Bd. 78, S. 694

1923. MARG. C. MANN. A demonstration of the stability of the genes of an inbred stock of Drosophila melano-gaster under experimental conditions. Journ. of exp. zoöl. Vol. 38, p. 213.

1919. O. MARBURG. Einige Probleme der Epileptiker Fürsorge. Wiener klin. Wochenschrift, 32. Jhrg., Nr. 9, S. 217.

1878. H. MARTIN. De la mortalité des enfants des épileptiques. Ann. méd. psych. 5e Sér. T. 19, p. 364.

1879. H. MARTIN. De l'alcoolisme des parents considéré comme cause d'épilepsie chez leurs descendants. Ann. méd. psychol. 6e sér., T. 1, 38e ann., p. 48.

1927 JOS. MAYER. Gesetzl. Unfruchtbarmachung Geisteskranker. Freiburg i. Br.

1914. W. MEDOW. Zur Erblichkeitsfrage in der Psychiatrie. Z. f. d. ges. Neur. u. Psych. 26. Bd., S. 493.

1911. L. MINOR. Zahlen und Beobachtungen aus dem Gebiete des Alkoholismus. Zeitschr. f. die ges. Neur. u. Psych., Bd. 4, S. 588.

1899. G. MIRTO. Sul potero terat. odeg. d. neur., d. alc. etil., etc. Ann. di neur., 27, 272. (cit. FÉRÉ).

1854. J. MOREAU de Tours. De l'étiologie de l'épilepsie. Mém. de l'acad. impér. de médec. T. 18.

1857. B. A. MOREL. Traité des dégénérescences physiques, intellectuelles et morales de l'espèce humaine. Paris. BAILLIÈRE.
MORGAN. The orientation of the frog's egg. Quarteïl. Journ. of microsc. science. Vol. 35, N. S.

1929. K. MOSER. Zur Frage der sog. selbstverschuldeten Trunkenheit, u.s.w. Arch. f. Psych. Bd. 86, S. 382.

1928. H. MUCKERMANN. Wirkungen des Alkoholgenusses auf die Nachkommenschaft. Berlin, Neuland Verlag, 1928.

1910. E. H. MÜLLER. Einige Beziehungen des Alkoholismus zur Aetiologie der Epilepsie. Monatschr. f. Psych. u. Neur. Bd. 28, Erg. H. p. 1.

1911. E. H. MÜLLER-SCHÜRCH. Der Alkoholismus als Ursache der Epilepsie. Epilepsia II, p. 333.

1910. E. MÜLLER. Demonstration aerztl. Ver. Marburg. M. m. W. N. 34, p. 1811.

1911 J. F. MUNSON. The Role of Heredity and other Factors in the Production of Traumatic Epilepsy. Epilepsia II, p. 343.

1924. L. J. J. MUSKENS. Epilepsie. Amsterdam. VAN ROSSEN (exists in Engl. transl.).

1908. P. NÄCKE. Die Zeugung im Rausche und ihre schädlichen Folgen für die Nachkommenschaft. Neur. Cent. Nr. 22.

1912. P. NÄCKE. Die Zeugung im Rausche und ihre schädlichen Folgen. Zeitschr. f. d. ges. Neur. u. Psych., Bd. 11, S. 218 (also D. med. W. 1913, N. 28, p. 1367).

1897. NEUMANN. Ueber die Beziehungen zwischen Alkoholismus und Epilepsie. Diss. Berlin. 1898. (cit. E. MÜLLER).

1912. L. B. NICE. Comparative Studies on the Effects of Alcohol, Nicotine, Tobacco Smoke and Caffeïne on White Mice. I. Effects on Reproduction and Growth. The Journ. of exper. zoöl. Vol. 12, p. 133.

1913. L. B. NICE. II. Effects on activity. Idem. Vol. 14, p. 123.

1917. L. B. NICE. Further observations on the effects of alcohol on white mice. American Naturalist. Vol. 51, p. 596.

1899. M. NICLOUX. Sur le passage de l'alcool ingéré par la mère au foetus, en particulier chez la femme, p. 980. C. r. soc. biol. Paris.

1899. M. NICLOUX. Sur le passage de l'alcool ingéré dans le lait chez la femme. Comptes rendus soc. biol., Paris, p. 982.

1900. M. NICLOUX. Sur le passage de l'alcool ingéré de la mère au foetus, etc. L'obstétrique, T. 5, p. 97.

1900. M. NICLOUX. Dosage comparatif de l'alcool, dans le sang et dans le lait, après ingestion dans l'estomac. Comptes rendus soc. biol. Paris, p. 295, 297, 620 et 622.

1928. J. NOTKIN. A contribution to the subject of epilepsy, with especial reference to the literature. Journ. of nerv. and ment. dis. Vol. 67, p. 321.

1908. H. OPPENHEIM. Lehrbuch der Nervenkrankheiten. Bd. II.

1927. OSTMANN. Beitrage zur Statistik der durch Alkohol hauptsächlich bedingten psychischen Erkrankungen. Allg. Zeitschr. f. Psych. 87. Bd, S., 243.

1928. OSTMANN. Gesammelte Notizen über unsere Epileptiker. Allg. Z. f. Psych. 89. Bd., S. 397

1929. PANSE. Alkohol u. Nachkommenschaft. Allg. Z. f. Psychiatr. 92, 72.

1916. R. PEARL. The effect of parental alcoholism (and certain other drug intoxications) upon the progeny in the domestic fowl. Proc. nat. acad. of science, Vol. 2, p. 380 and 675.

1916. R. PEARL. On the effect of continued administration of certain poisons to the domestic fowl, with special reference to the progeny. Proc. Amer. Phil. Soc. Vol. 45, p. 243, meeting of April 15th.

1917. R. PEARL. The experimental modification of germ cells. I. General plan of experiments with ethyl alcohol and certain related substances, p. 125, Vol. 22, II. The effect upon the domestic fowl of the daily inhalation of ethyl alcohol and certain related substances, p. 165. III. The effect of parental alcoholism and certain other drug intoxications upon the progeny, p. 24. The Journal exp. Zoöl. Vol. 22.

1924. R. PEARL. The racial effect fo alcohol. Eugenics Review. April.

1930. R. PEARL. Alcohol. Biological Aspects. In The Encyclopaedia of social sciences. Vol. 1. Macmillan Co.

1930. R. PEARL. Requirements of a proof that natural selection has altered a race. Scientia, mars 1930, p. 175.

1925. R. PEARL and AGN. ALLEN. The influence of alcohol upon the growth of seedlings. Journ. Gen. Physiol. Vol. 8, p. 215.

1910. K. PEARSON. On a new method of determining correlation. Biometrika. 7, 248.

1910. K. PEARSON and E. M. ELDERTON. A first study of the influence of parental alcoholism, etc. Eugenics Laboratory Memoirs X, 2nd ed.

1910. K. PEARSON and E. M. ELDERTON. A second study, etc. Being a reply.

1911. KARL PEARSON. Erwiderung auf die Notiz von Dr. ALLERS über die Trinkenkinder. Arch. f. Rass. u. Ges.biol. 8. Jhrg. S. 377.

1927. E. PFEIFER. Einfluss der Diurese auf den Alkoholgehalt des Blutes, Pharmak. Beitrage zur Alkoholfrage, H. 3, Jena.

1912. PFÖRRINGER. Tierversuche über den erbl. Einfluss des Alkohols. Allg. Zeitschr. für Psychiatrie u.s.w. 69, 734.

1924. A. PICTET. Résultats négatifs d'expériences d'alcoolisme sur les Cobayes. etc. C.r. Soc. de physique et d'hist. nat. de Genève 41, 29.

1924. A. PICTET. Actions des vapeurs d'alcool éthylique sur le développement et la pigmentation des Lépidoptères. C. r. Soc. de phys. et d'hist. nat. Genève 41, 33.

1928. A. PILCZ. Die weiteren Lebensschicksale von Kindern, welche während des Bestehens einer mütterlichen Geistes- oder Nervenkrankheit geboren worden sind. (2. Mitt.) Jahrb. f. Psych. u. Neur. 46, 113.

1903. A. PLOETZ. Der Alkohol im Lebensprozess der Rasse. Bericht über das 9. int. Kon. gress gegen den Alkohol, Bremen. Apr. 1903, S. 70.

1927a. K. POLISCH. Die Persönlichkeit und das Milieu Delirium-tremens. Kranker der Charité aus den Jahren 1912—1925. Monatschr. f. Psych. u. Neur. Bd. 63, S. 136.

1927b. K. POLISCH. Die pathogenetische Bedeutung der Gelegenheitsursachen für das Delirium-tremens. Monatschr. f. Psych. u. Neur. Bd. 63, S. 69.

1927c. K. POLISCH. Die Nachkommenschaft Delirium-tremens. Kranker, (Ein Beitrag zur Frage. Alkohol und Keimschädigung). Monatschr. f. Psych. u. Neur. Bd. 64, S. 108 u. 373.

1929. K. POLISCH. Alkohol u. Nachkommenschaft. Int. Z. Alk. H. 6, p. 14.

1930. K. POLISCH. Alkohol. Fortschr. Neur. Psych. II, 417.

1918. H. PREISIG und K. AMADIAN (MAHAIM). Les alcooliques sont-ils des dégénérés? Schweiz. Arch. f. Neur. u. Psych. Bd. 3, p. 147, (also: Arch f. Neur. u. Psych. II, p. 355).

1914. E. Redlich. Statistisches zur Aetiologie der Nerven- und Geistes-krankheiten. Wiener klin. Wochenschrift Nr. 44, S. 1419.

1923. E. Redlich. Epilepsie. Lewandowsky's Handb. d. Neurol. Suppl. Bd., S. 407.

1921. H. Reiter u. H. Osthoff. Die Bedeutung endogener und exogener Faktoren bei Kindern der Hilfsschule. Zeitschr. f. Hyg. 94, 224.

1925. Th. Ribot. L'Hérédité psychologique. 11me éd. Paris, p. 92—94.

1904. S. P. Rietema. Tuberculose en erfelijkheid. Ned. Tijdschr. voor Geneesk. I, blz. 108.

1912. G. H. Roger. Les Intoxications. In Bouchart en Roger. T. II, p. 1.

1922. Roger, Widal, Teissier. Nouveau traité de médecine. Fasc VI. G. H. Roger. Les Intoxications.

1921. Romeis, communicated in Bilski, 1921.

1914. J. Rosenberg (pseudoniem) Familien-Degeneration und Alkohol. Die Amberger im XIX. Jahrhundert. Zeitschr. f. d. ges. Neur. u. Psych. Bd. 22, S. 133—240.

1925. E. Rost und G. Wolf. Zur Frage der Beeinflussung der Nachkom-menschaft durch den Alkohol im Tierversuch. Arch. f. Hyg. 95. Bd., S. 140.

1903. E. Rüdin. Der Alkohol im Lebensprozess der Rasse. Bericht über das 9. int. Kongress gegen den Alkohol, Bremen. April 1903, S. 95.

1905. E. Rüdin. Ergänzende Bemerkungen zu O. Diem's Artikel u.s.w. Arch. f. Rass. u. Ges. Biol. Bd. 2, S. 470.

1916. E. Rüdin. Zur Vererbung und Neuentstehung der Dementia Preacox. Monogr. a. d. ges. Geb. der Neur. u. Psych., Julius Springer, Berlin.

1924. E. Rüdin. Der gegenwärtige Stand der Epilepsieforschung. Zeitschr. f. d. ges. Neur. u. Psych. Bd. 89, S. 374 u. 375.

1924. E. Rüdin. Erblichkeit und Psychiatrie. Zeitschr. f. d. ges. Neur. u. Psych. 93, 502.

1906. Th. Rybakow. Alkoholismus und Erblichkeit. Monatschr. f. Neur. u. Psych. XX, 221.

1920. K. Schaffer. Die allgemeine histopathologische Charakterisierung der Heredo-degeneration. Schweiz. Archiv f. Neur. u.Psych.Bd. 7, p.193.

1924. R. Schinz u. B. Slotopolsky. Beitr. z. exper. Path. d. Hodens, usw. Denkschr d. Schweiz. nat. forsch. Ges. 61, 29. (Lit.).

1913. E. Schlesinger. Das psychische Verhalten der schwachbegabten Schulkinder und ihre Characterentwicklung. Zeitschr. f. d. ges. Neur. u. Psych. Bd. 17, S. 10.

1912. H. Schotmüller und O. Schumm. Nachweis von Alkohol in der Spi-nalflüssigkeit von Säufern. Neur. Cent. 1021.

1913. H. Schotmüller und O. Schumm. Ueber den Nachweis von Alkohol in der Spinalflüssigkeit von Säufern. Zeitschr. f. d. ges. Neur. u. Psych. Bd. 15, p. 634.

1926. G. Schreiber, D. Reich u. D. Mediz. Stud. z. med. pol. d. R. in der Nachkriegszeit (1918—1926). cit. Jos. Mayer.

1912. P. SCHRÖDER. Diskussion zu PFÖRRINGER. Allg. Zeitschr. f. Psychiatrie u.s.w. 69, 734.

1913. P. SCHRÖDER. Versuche mit chronischer Alkoholintoxikation bei Kaninchen. Monatschr. f. Psychiatrie und Neurologie. Bd. 34, S. 1.

1906—1907. E. SCHWALBE. Die Morphologie der Missbildungen. I. Teil. Allgemeine Missbildungslehre. Jena.

1911. E. SCHWALBE. Allgemeine Pathologie. Stuttgart.

1926. SCHWEIGHÖFER. Die Familie 135. Eine sozialpsychiatrische Untersuchung. Zeitschr. f. d. ges. Neur. u. Psych. Bd. 104, S. 623.

1910. M. SICHEL. Der Alkohol als Ursache der Belastung. Neur. Cent. p. 738 29. Jhrg.

1898. M. SIMMONDS. Die Ursachen der Azoospermie. Deutsch-Arch. f. Klin. Med. 61, 412.

1910. M. SIMMONDS. Ueb. Fibrosis-testis. Arch. f path. anat. (Virchow) 201, 108 (Also Berl. Kl. W. 35, 70, 1911).

1925. J. CHR. SMITH. Arvelighed og Alkohol. Inledning af W. JOHANNSEN, Kobenhavn. J. H. SCHULTZ.

1921. O. SNELL. Die Belastungsverhältnisse bei der genuïnen Epilepsie. Zeitschr. f. d. ges. Neur. u. Psych. 70. Bd, S. 1.

1914. G. STEINER. Ueber die familiäre Anlage zur Epilepsie. Zeitschr. f. d. ges. Neur. und Psych. 23. Bd., S. 315.

1923. H. STIEVE. Der Einfluss des Alkohols auf die Samenbildung der Hausmaus. Nat. Wis. Korz. Bd. 1. (cit. Stieve).

1910. CH. R. STOCKARD. The influence of alcohol and other anaesthetics on embryonic development. The American Journal of Anatomy. Vol. 10, p. 369.

1912. CH. R. STOCKARD. An experimental study of racial degeneration in mammals treated with alcohol. The archives of internal medicine. Vol. X, p. 369. (lit.)

1913. CH. R. STOCKARD. The effect on the offspring of intoxicating the male parent and the transmission of the defects to subsequent generations. American Naturalist, 47, 641.

1913. CH. R. STOCKARD and DOROTHY M. CRAIG. An experimental study of the influence of alcohol on the germ cells and the developing embryos of mammals. Arch. f. Entw. mech. Bd. 35, p. 569.

1916. CH. R. STOCKARD and G. PAPANICOLAOU. A further analysis of the hereditary transmission of degeneracy and deformities by the descendants of alcoholized mammals. American Naturalist 50, p. 65.

1918. CH. R. STOCKARD and G. PAPANICOLAOU. Further studies on the modifications of the germ cells in mammals. The effect of alcohol on treated guinea-pigs and their descendants. Journ. exper. Zoöl. Vol. 26, p. 119.

1922. CH. R. STOCKARD. Alcohol as a selective agent in the improvement of racial stock. The Brit. med. Journ. N. 3215, p. 255.

1924. CH. R. STOCKARD. Alcohol a factor in eliminating racial degeneracy. Amer. Journal of the med. science. Vol. 167, p. 469.

1901. W. Strohmayer. Ueber die Bedeutung der Individualstatistik bei der Erblichkeitsfrage in der Neuro- und Psychopathologie. Münch. med. Woch. Nr. 45, S. 1786 u. 1842.

1908. W. Strohmayer. Zur Kritik der Feststellung und der Bewertung psychoneur. erbl. Belastung. Arch. f. Rass. u. Ges. Biol. p. 478.

1910. W. Strohmayer. Vorlesung. Psychopathologie des Kindesalters. Tübingen.

1913. W. Strohmayer. Die Bedeutung des Mendelismus für die klin. Vererbungslehre. Fortschr. d. Deutschen Klin. 3. Bd., S. 331.

1928. W. Strohmayer. Angeborene Schwachsinnzustände. In O. Bumke, Hndb. d. Geisteskrankh. X. Spez. VI.

1921. Stüber. Die erbliche Belastung bei der Epilepsie. Zent. f. d. ges. Neur. u. Psych. Bd. 25, S. 361.

1915. J. Stüchlik. Ueber die hereditären Beziehungen zwischen Alkoholismus und Epilepsie. Corr.-Blatt für Schweizer Aerzte, 45, 70.

1900. W. Ch. Sullivan. The children of the female drunkard. The med. temp. Rev. III, p. 72.

1877. H. Taguet. De l'hérédité dans l'alcoolisme. Ann. méd. psych. 5e sér. t. 18.

1919. N. Ph. Tendeloo. Allgemeine Pathologie. Julius Springer, Berlin.

1915. D. A. Thom. The relation between the genetic factors etc. of hered. epilepsy. Boston med. and surg. Journ. 173, p. 469.

1916a. D. A. Thom. The frequency of epilepsy in the offspring of epileptics. Boston med. and surg. journ. 174, p. 573.

1916b. D. A. Thom. A second note on the frequency of epilepsy in the offspring of epileptics. Boston med. and surg. Journ. 175, p. 599.

1907. Tigges. Untersuchungen über die erblich belasteten Geisteskranken. Allg. Zeitschr. f. Psychiatrie. Bd. 64, S. 1 u. 891.

1921. Tilmann. Zur Pathogenese der Epilepsie. Virchow's Archiv, 40, 229.

1910. C. Todde. L'azione dell' alcool sullo sviluppo e sulla funsione dei testicoli. Riv. sper. di Freniatria. 36, 491. N. 31.

1891. E. Toulouse. Convulsions infantiles par alcoolisme de la nourrice. Gazette des Hopitaux, No. 98, p. 914.

1896. E. Toulouse. Les causes de la folie, Paris.

1922. H. Triboulet et R. Mignot. L'alcoolisme p. 247. Masson & Cie Paris.

1911. W. A. Turner. The problem of epilepsy. Elepsia II p. 23.

1926. G. Vacca. Ricerche sulle alteraz. testic. nell'avelenamento sperim. da caffeina. Arch. Pharm. sper. 42, 62. (cit. Bluhm).

1872. Vernay. Convulsions par alcool chez un nouveau-né, Lyon médical, Nov. 1872.

1928. E. J. Verwey. Alkohol en nageslacht. Academia-Verh. met inl. v. Prof. K. H. Bouman. De Wegwijzer 29, 1, p. 41.

1926. Vieilledent. Dosage de l'alcool dans le sang et diagnostie de l'ivresse Gaz. d. hôp. vic. et mil. Ann. 99. Nr. 53, p. 853. Ref. Zent. f. d. Ges. Neur. u. Psych. 45, 153, 1927.

1910. H. Vogt. Die Epilepsie im Kindesalter. Berlin.

1883. A. Voisin. Leçons clin. sur les maladies mentales, etc. Paris.

1897. Jules Voisin. L'epilepsie. Paris.

1930. Het Volkenbondsonderzoek naar de oorzaken der zuigelingensterfte. Leiden.

1914. Volland. Histologische Untersuchungen bei epileptischen Krankheitsbildern. I. Z. f. d. ges. Neur. und Psych. Bd. 21, S. 195.

1913. Vorkästner und Neue. Ueber den Nachweis von Alkohol in der Spinalflüssigkeit von Säufern. Z. f. d. ges. Neur. u. Psych. Bd. 14, S. 324.

1911. B. H. Vos. Verschiedene Gesichtspunkte über den Zusammenhang zwischen Alkoholismus und Tuberkulose. Monatschr. z. Erforsch. v. Alkoh. u.s.w. Nr. 12, 1911.

1917. E. de Vries. De lichamelijke constitutie van den mensch. De toekomst der maatschappij. Wereld-Bibliotheek, Amsterdam.

1928. J. Wagner-Jauregg. Ueber Erblichkeit in der Pathologie. Wien. Kl. Woch. Nr. 16 u. 17, S. 545 u. 595.

1928. H. Wegener. Der gegenwärtige Stand des Alkoholismus nach dem Material der rheinischen Provinzialanstalten. Archiv. für Psych. Bd. 85, S. 281.

1912. A. Weichselbaum und J. Kyrle. Ueber die Veränderungen der Hoden bei chronischem Alkoholismus, S. 51. Sitz. ber. Königl. Acad. der Wiss., Wien. Nat. Cl. Abt. 3, Bd. 120; ook Bd. 121, S. 51.

1918. W. Weinberg. Künstliche Fehlgeburt und künstliche Unfruchtbarkeit vom Standpunkt der Statistik. Placzek's Jandb. f. künstl. Fehlgeb. u. künstl. Unfr. Leipzig, 1918. S. 437.

1928. G. Weise. Ueber die erbliche Belastung in Fällen von sogen. traumatischer Epilepsie im Vergleich mit solcher von sogen. genuïner Epilepsie. Arch. f. Psych. 85, 248.

1930. C. V. Weller. Degenerative changes in the male germinalepithelium in acute alcoholism and their possible relationship to blastophthoria. Amer. J. Path. N. 1, p. 1. (cit. Bluhm).

1897. Wildermath. Alkohol, Trauma u. Epilepsie. Z. f. Behandl. Schwachs. u. Epil. Ref. Neur. Cent., p. 703.

1911. R. A. Witthaus. Manual of Toxicology. 2nd Ed. London, 1911.

1929. R. Wlassak. Grundriss der Alkoholfrage. 2. verm. Aufl. Hirzel, Leipzig.

1907. R. Wolfsohn. Die Heredität bei Dementia praecox. Allg. Z. f. Psych. Bd. 64 S. 347.

1913. M. Woods. Seven Cases of Epilepsy in Children. The Amer. Journ. med. Assoc. Vol. 61, p. 2291.

1921. J. Wyrsch. Zur Frage der geographischen Verbreitung und polyklinischen Therapie der Epilepsie. Arch. f. Neur. u. Psych. Bd. 9, S. 309.

B. The other germ poisons

1914. L. ADLER. Ueber Jodschädigungen der Hoden. Arch. f. expérim. Path. u. Pharm. 75, 362.

1894. M. ANKER. Ein Fall von wahrscheinlich hereditärer Bleilähmung. Berl. klin. Woch. Nr. 25, p. 577.

1894. B. ANNINO. Avvelenamento cronico da piombo. Arch. ital. di Clin. med. 32, 4, p. 72. Lavore sperimentale. (ref. in VIRCHOW-HIRSCH'S Jahresber. üb. 1894.

1908. ARCICHOVSKIJ. Z. Frage über den Einfluss v. ZnSO₄ auf eine Reihe von Generationen von Aspergillus niger. Cent. f. Bakt. Abt. II, Bd. 21, 1908, S. 430.

1928. E. W. BAADER. Die Erkennung der chronischen Bleivergiftung. Zeitschr. für ärztl. Fortb. p. 205.

1927. G. BAKACS. Exper. weibl. Genitaltuberkulose. Arch. f. Gyn. 131, 364.

1920. F. M. BALDWIN. Susceptible and resistant phases of the dividing sea-urchin egg, when subjected to various concentrations of lipoidsoluble substances, especially the higher alcohols. Biol. Bull. Vol. 38, p. 123.

1894. W. BATESON. Materials for the study of Variation. London.

1929. BAUR. Auslösung neuer erblicher Eigensch. durch starke physikalische u. chemische Reize. M. med. W. Nr. 51, S. 2157.

1874. BERGER. Ein Beitrag zur Lehre von der Encephalopathia saturnina. Berl. klin. Woch. Nr. 11 u. 12.

1908. W. H. BLOEMENDAL. Arsenicum in het dierlijk organisme. Diss. med. Leiden.

1902. BROUARDEL. Les empoisonnements, p. 433.

1922. A. BUSCHKE und B. PEISER. Die Wirkung des Thallium auf das endokrine System. Klin. Woch. 1 Jahrg. Nr. 20, S. 995.

1927. A. BUSCHKE und BERMANN. Weitere Untersuchungen über die Wirkung von Metallsalzen auf den Brunstzyklus der Maus. M. m. W. 74. Jahrg. Nr. 23, S. 969. Zie ook: Klin. Woch. 1917, Nr. 15 en Arch. f. Dermat. 1908.

1914. L. J. COLE and L. J. BACHHUBER. The effect of lead on the germ cells of the small rabbit and fowl as indicated by their progeny. Proc. Soc. f. exper. biol. and med. Vol. XII, p. 24.

1907. S. CONNATA. Tabagismo e funzioni genetali nell' uomo, Gazz. degli ospedali e delle cliniche. Milan, 28, 910. N. 87 (cit. NICE).

1911. S. CROCE. Ueber den Einfluss natürlicher Arsenwässer und künstlicher Arsenlösungen auf den Stoffwechsel. Zeitschr. f. klin. Medizin. Bd. 37, S. 103.

1928. E. CZARNECKI et I. JOLLY Action des rayons ultraviolets sur le testicule. Comptes-rendus soc. biol., Paris, 98, 1928, 5, p. 380.

1891. C. DARESTE. Recherches sur la production artificielle des monstruosités, 2me ed. Paris.

1893. C. Dareste. Note sur l'influence des vapeurs mercurielles sur le développement de l'embryon. C. r. soc. biol., Paris, p. 683.

1924. 1927. W. E. Dixon. Nicotin in A. Heffter's Handb. der exper. Pharmakologie. S. 658. 2. Bd., 2. Hälfte. III, 1, p. 680. Springer, Berlin.

1909. P. Ehrlich. Beitrage zur exper. Path. u. Chemotherapie Leipzig 1909 u. in and. Schriften.

1928. J. M. Evvard. Jodine deficiency symptoms etc. Endocrinology, 12, 539.

1893. Ch. Féré. Note sur l'influence de la lumière blanche et de la lumière colorée sur l'incubation des oeufs de la poule. C. r. soc. biol. Paris p. 745 et 944.

1893. Ch. Féré. Note sur l'influence de l'éthérisation préalable sur l'incubation des oeufs de la poule. C.r. soc. viol. Paris p. 749.

1893. Ch. Féré. Note sur l'influence de l'exposition préalable aux vapeurs d'alcool sur l'incubation de l'oeuf de la poule. C. r. soc. biol., Paris, p. 773.

1893. Ch. Féré. Note sur l'influence des injections de liquide dans l'albumen sur l'incubation de l'oeuf de la poule. C. r. soc. biol. Paris, p. 787.

1893. Ch. Féré. Note sur l'incubation de l'oeuf de poule, d'injections préalables dans l'albumen de solutions de sel, de glucose, de glycerine. C.r. s.b. Paris, p. 831.

1893. Ch. Féré. Note sur l'influence de l'exposition préalable aux vapeurs de chloroforme sur l'incubation des oeufs de poule. C.r. s.b. Paris, p. 849.

1893. Ch. Féré. Note sur l'influence de l'exposition préalable aux vapeurs d'essence de térébenthine sur l'incubation des oeufs de poule. C. r. s. b., Paris, p. 852.

1893. Ch. Féré. Note sur l'influence de l'exposition préalable aux vapeurs des essences sur l'incubation des oeufs de poule. C. r. s. b., Paris, p. 945.

1893. Ch. Féré. Note sur l'influence de l'exposition préalable á la fumée de tabac et aux vapeur de nicotine, sur l'incubation des oeufs de poule, p. 948

1894. Ch. Féré. Action tératogène de l'alcool méthylique. C. r. s. b., Paris, p. 221.

1894. Ch. Féré. Influence tératogène des isoalcools.

1894. Ch. Féré. Vapeurs mercurielles. Leur action sur le développement de l'embryon de poulet. C. r. s. b. Paris, p. 282.

1894. Ch. Féré. Note sur l'influence des enduits partiels sur l'incubation de l'oeuf de poule. C. r. s. b., Paris, p. 63.

1894. Ch. Féré. Expériences sur la puissance tératogène ou dégénérative des alcools dits supérieurs. Bull. et mém. d. l. Soc. méd. des hôp., p. 136 (cit. Féré).

1894. Ch. Féré. Notes sur les différences des effets des agents toxiques et des vibrations mécaniques sur l'évolution de l'embryon de poulet suivant l'époque où elles agissent. C. r. soc. biol., Paris, p. 462.

1894. Ch. Féré. Note sur la résistance de l'embryon de poulet à certaines toxines microbiennes introduites dans l'albumen de l'oeuf. C. r. soc. biol., Prais, p. 490.

1894. CH. FÉRÉ. Note sur l'influence de la déshydration sur le développement de l'embryon de poulet. C. r. soc. biol., Paris, p. 614.

1894. CH. FÉRÉ. Présentation de poulets vivants provenant d'oeufs ayant subi des injections d'alcool éthylique dans l'albumen. C. r. soc. biol., Paris, p. 646.

1894. CH. FÉRÉ. Note sur la coexistence fréquente des arrêts de développement du bec supérieur et des anomalies de la tête chez l'embryon du poulet. C. r. soc. biol., Paris, p. 719.

1895. CH. FÉRÉ. De l'influence de la nicotine injectée dans l'albumen sur l'incubation de l'oeuf de poule. C. r. soc. biol., Paris, p. 11.

1895. CH. FÉRÉ. Notes sur les effets différents sur l'évolution de l'embryon de poulet d'une même substance, suivant les doses. C. r. soc. biol., Paris, p. 673.

1895. CH. FÉRÉ. Note sur l'influence de l'exposition préalable des oeufs de poule aux vapeurs de phosphore sur l'évolution de l'embryon. C. r. soc. biol., Paris, p. 677.

1896. CH. FÉRÉ. Faits relatifs de la tendance á la variation sous l'influence de changements de milieu. C. r. soc. biol. p. 790.

1896. CH. FÉRÉ. Note sur l'influence des injections de la solution dite physiol de sel, etc. C. r. soc. biol., p. 938.

1896. CH. FÉRÉ. Recherches sur la puissance tératogène et sur la puissance toxique de l'acétone. Arch. de phys. norm. et path., 6e sér. t. 8, p. 239 et 341 (cit. FÉRÉ).

1896. CH. FÉRÉ. Note sur l'influence des injections de peptone dans l'albumen de l'oeuf de poule sur l'évolution de l'embryon. C. R. Soc. biol. Paris. p. 424.

1898. CH. FÉRÉ. Note sur l'influence de l'injection préalable de solutions de créatine dans l'albumen de l'oeuf etc. C. R. Soc. biol. Paris, p. 499.

1898. CH. FÉRÉ. Note sur l'influence de l'injection préalable de solutions de xanthocréatine dans l'albumen de l'oeuf etc. C. R. Soc. biol. Paris, p. 711.

1899. CH. FÉRÉ. Influence de l'injection préalable de bromure de potassium, etc. C. r. s. b. p. 713.

1899. CH. FÉRÉ. Influence du repos sur les effets de l'exposition préalable aux vapeurs d'alcool avant l'incubation, etc. C. r. s. b. p. 255

1899. CH. FÉRÉ. Note sur l'influence de l'exposition préalable aux vapeurs d'ammoniaque, etc. C. r. s. b. p. 806.

1899. CH. FÉRÉ. Note sur la tolérance de l'embryon de poulet pour l'iodure de potassium. C. r. s. b., Paris, p. 454.

1900. CH. FÉRÉ. Note sur l'influence des injections préalables de solutions de caféine dans l'albumen de l'oeuf sur l'évolution de l'embryon de poulet. C. r. s. b., Paris, p. 471.

1900. CH. FÉRÉ. Note sur l'influence des injections préalables de solutions de cantharidine dans l'albumen de l'oeuf sur l'évolution de l'embryon de poulet. C. r. soc. biol. Par. p. 681.

1900. CH. FÉRÉ. Note sur l'influence de l'échauffement préalables sur l'incubation de l'oeuf de poule. C. r. soc. biol., Paris, p. 796.

1900. CH. FÉRÉ. Note sur la multiplicité des causes des variations de l'orientation de l'embryon de poulet. Journ. anat. Phys. 36, 210.

1929. R. FETSCHER. Erblichkeit erworbener Eigensch. Die Umschau 33, H. 7.

1908. C. FLEIG. Influence de la fumée de tabac et de la nicotine sur le développement de l'organisme. C. r. soc. biol., Paris, Ann.1908, T. 1, p. 683

1872. A. P. FOKKER. Over den invloed van arsenicum op de stofwisseling. Ned. Tijdschr. voor Geneesk. 2e reeks, 8e jaarg., 1e afl., blz. 1.

1929. A. FORSTER. Versuche über den Einfluss der chronischen Bleivergiftung auf den Vaginalzyklus der Ratte. Endokrinologie. 4, 1929, 4, S. 260,

1926. FRIEDBERGER. Ausspräche zu FÜRBRINGER. Zur Würdigung der Gefahren des Tabakrauchens. Münch. med. Wochenschr. Nr. 46, S. 1956.

1836. Is. GEOFFROY ST. HILAIRE. Hist. gén. et part. de l'organisation chez l'homme et les animaux. Paris. 3 Vol. et atl.

1925. H. GILFORD. Tumors and Cancers. London. Selwijn and Bount (cit. Bluhm).

1928. P. GLEY. Modifications histologiques du tractus génital femelle sous l'action de l'hormone du corps jaune. Comptes rendus soc. biol., Paris, 98, 11, p. 834.

1929. R. GOLDSCHMIDT. Experimentelle Mutation und das Problem der sogenannten Parallelinduktion. Versuche an Drosophila. Biol. Cent. 49, S. 437.

1907. K. GRASSMANN. Über Einfluss des Nikotins auf die Zirkulation. Münch. med. Woch. 1907, S. 975.

1922. J. GUGGENHEIMER. Lebensfähigkeit der menschl. Spermien. Monatschr. Gynaek. 59, 1922.

1907. G. GÜNTHER. Ueber Spermiengifte. PFLÜGER's Arch. 118, S. 551.

1920. GUYER and SMITH. Studies on cytolysins. II. Transmission of induced eye-defects. Journ. of exp. zoöl. 31, 171.

1930. F. B. HANSON and E. WINKLEMAN. Visible mutations following radium irradiation in Drosophila melanogaster. Journ. of Heredity 20, 277.

1921. A. HARTMANN. Ueber die Einwirkung von Röntgenstrahlen auf Amphibienlarven. Arch. f. Entw. mech. 47, 135.

1927. R. HATCHER and H. CROSBY. Journ. of Pharmac. 32.

1928. F. HECKE. Die Thalliumvergiftung und ihre histologischen Veränderungen bei Ratten. VIRCHOW's Archiv. Bd. 269, I. H., S. 28 und 29.

1923—1927. A. HEFFTER. Handb. d. exper. Pharmakologie. JUL. SPRINGER, Berlin. 1. u. 2. Bd., 3. Bd., 1. H.

1927. A. HEFFTER und E. KEESER. Arsen und seine Verbindungen. III, 1, 463, 1927.

HERBST. Exper. Unters. über den Einfluss der veränd. chem. Zusammensetz. d. umgeb. Med. auf die Entw. d. Tiere. Mitt. zoöl. Station Neapel. Bd. XI (cit. O. HERTWIG).

1911. G. HERTWIG. Radiumbestrahlung unbefruchteter Froscheier u. ihre Entw. nach Befr. m. norm. Samen. Arch. f. mikr. Anat. 77 II. Abt. 165.

1913. G. und P. HERTWIG. Beeinflussung der männlichen Keimzellen durch chemische Stoffe. Arch. f. mikr. Anat. 2 Abt. 83. Bd., S. 267.

1887. O. und R. HERTWIG. Ueber den Befruchtungs- und Teilungsvorgang des tierischen Eies unter dem Einfluss äusserer Agentien. In: Untersuchungen zur Morph. u. Phys. d. Zelle von O. u. R. HERTWIG. H. 5, Jena.

1892. O. HERTWIG. Urmund und Spina bifida. Eine vgl. morph. teratol. Studie an missgebildeten Froscheiern. Arch. f. mikr. Anat. 39, S. 353.

1895. O. HERTWIG. Beitr. zur exper. Morphol. und Entwickl. gesch. Die Entwicklung des Froscheies unter dem Einfluss schwäch. u. stärk. Kochsalzlösungen. Arch. f. mikr. Anat. 44. Bd., S. 285.

1896. O. HERTWIG. Exper. Erzeugungen tierischer Missbildungen. Festschr. f. Gegenbaur. 2. B., S. 87.

1911. O. HERTWIG. Die Radiumkrankheit tierischer Keimzellen. Arch. f. mikr. Anat. 77, II. Abt., S. 1—165.

1912. O. HERTWIG. Veränderung der idioplasmatischen Beschaffenheit der Samenfäden durch physikalische und durch chemische Eingriffe. Sitz. ber. Königl. Preuss. Akad. der Wiss. 1912, XXXI, S. 554.

1912. O. HERTWIG. Allgemeine Biologie. 4. Auflage. Jena.

1913. O. HERTWIG. Keimesschädigung durch chemische Eingriffe. Sitz. ber. phys. math. Cl. Königl. Preuss. Akad. d. Wissensch. Jahrg.1913, I, S. 564.

1917. PAULA HERTWIG. Beeinflussung der Geschlechtszellen und der Nachkommensch. durch Bestrahlung mit radioaktiven Substanzen. Zeitschr. f. ind. Abst. u. Vererb.l. 17, S. 254.

1918. PAULA HERTWIG. Keimesschädigung durch physikalische und chemische Eingriffe. Zeitschr. f. ind. Abst.- und Vererb.l. 19, S. 79.

1927. PAULA HERTWIG. Partielle Keimesschädigungen durch Radium und Röntgenstrahlen. Handbuch der Vererbungswissensch. Bd. III, Lf. 1 (III, A. u. C.). E. BAUR und R. HARTMANN.

1918. M. A. VAN HERWERDEN. Untersuchungen über die parthenogenetische und geschlechtliche Fortpflanzung von Daphnia pulex. Verh. Kon. Acad. der Wetensch. 2e sect. Dl. 20, N. 3.

1919. M. A. VAN HERWERDEN. De invloed van radiumstralen op de ontwikkeling der eieren van Daphnia pulex. Genetica. Dl. 1, p. 305.

1908. G. HERXHEIMER und K. F. HOFFMANN. Ueber die anatomischen Wirkungen der Röntgenstrahlen auf den Hoden. Deutsche med. Woch. Nr. 36, p. 1551.

1927. HODGSON, VARDON, SINGH. Studies on the effects of antimony salts. N. 1. The effect of antimony salts on conception and pregnancy in animals. Indian Journ. med. Res. 15(2), 491—495, 1927. (Ref. Biol. Abstr. Vol. 2, N. 1—5, 1928).

1923. R. Hofstätter. Experimentelle Studie über die Einwirkung des Nico-
tins auf die Keimdrüsen und auf die Fortpflanzung. Virchow's Arch.,
Bd. 244, S. 183.

1920. Jaschke u. Pankow. Lehrb. d. Geburtshilfe p. 317.

1923. Joël. Kokaïnismus. Mediz. Ges., Berlin. Deutsche med. Wochenschr.
Nr. 9, S. 295.

1926. W. Johannsen. Elemente der exakten Erblichkeitslehre. 3. Aufl.
Jena.

1902. L. Jorès. Ueber die pathologische Anatomie der chronischen Bleivergiftung des Kaninchens. Ziegler's Beitr. zur pathol. Anat., Bd. 31,
S. 183.

1926. K. Kawamoto. Hodenuntersuchungen bei verschiedenen Erkrankungen, insbesondere Cholesterinämien. Frankf. Zeit. f. Path. Bd. 34, S.409,

1910. H. B. Koldewijn. Overgang van geneesmiddelen in melk. Diss., Leiden.

1856. A. Kölliker. Physiologische Studien. üb. die Samenflüssigkeit
Zeitschr. f. Wiss. zool. 7, 201. (oude litt.).

1926. A. Kostitch and A. Telebakovitch. Jodine. C. r. Soc. biol. Paris 94,
986 (cit. Kostitch et V.).

1927. Kostitch et Verbitzki. De l'action blastophthorique de l'arsenic.
C. r. d. l. Soc. biol. de Paris (de Belgrade) p. 999.

1929. Kräuter. Ueber die Einwirkung von Giften auf den fötalen Organismus. Schweiz. med. Woch. 1929. N. 46, S. 1165.

1928. A. E. Kulkow. Eigenartige Besonderheiten der Quecksilberencepha-
lopathie. Zeitschr. für die ges. Neur. u. Psych., 116, S. 780.

1861. A. A. Kussmaul. Unters. üb. d. constit. Mercurialismus. Würzburg.

1872. A. Kussmaul und R. Maier. Zur pathol. Anatomie des chronischen
Saturnismus. Deutsches Archiv f. klin. Med. 9. Bd.

1889. H. Legrand et L. Winter. Un cas de saturnisme héréditaire. C. r.
d. l. Soc. de Biol. 1889, p. 46.

1908. Lehmann. Unters. über das Tabakrauchen. Münch. med. Woch.
1908, S. 723. (Ref. Arch. f. Rass. u. Ges. Biol. 1908, S. 577).

1916. Lemkes. Dissertatie, Leiden.

1899. L. Lewin. Ueber eigentumliche Quecksilberanwendungen. Berl. klin.
Wochenschrift Nr. 13, S. 276, 356 en 376 (Bleipfläster als Abortivum).

J. Loeb. Experiments on cleavage. Journ. Morph. 7.

1895. J. Loeb. Die chemische Entwicklungserregung des tierischen Eies.
Pflüger's Archiv. Bd. 62.

1896. J. Loeb. Untersuchungen über die physiol. Wirkungen des Sauer-
stoffmangels. Pflüger's Archiv. Bd. 62, S. 249.

1903. Jacques Loeb. Ueber die Befruchtung von Seeïgeleiern durch See-
sternsamen. Arch. f. d. ges. Phys. 99, S. 323.

1907. J. Loeb. Ueber die allgemeinen Methoden der künstl. Parthenogenese.
Pflüger's Arch. 181, S. 575.

1917. L. Loeb. The experimental production of hypotypical ovaries through underfeeding. A contribution to the analysis of sterility. Biol. Bull. Vol. 33, p. 91.

1914. O. LOEB und B. ZÖPPRITZ. Die Beeinflussung der Fortpflanzungs-fähigkeit durch Jod. Deutsche med. Woch. Nr. 25, S. 1261.

1914. D. T. MAC DOUGAL. The effect of potassium iodide, methyleneblue and other substances applied to the embryo sacs of seed-plants. Proc. Soc. Exp. Biol. Med. 12, p. 1.

1882. R. MAIER. Experimentelle Studien über Bleivergiftung. I. VIRCHOW's Archiv, Bd. 90, S. 455.

1900. S. METALNIKOFF. Etudes sur la spermatoxine. Ann. de l'Inst. PASTEUR, 14e année, No. 9, p. 577.

1854. A. MILLET. Du seigle ergoté cons. s. l. rapp. physiol., obstétr., etc. Mém. acad. impér. de méd. T. 18, p. 283, Paris.

1906. D. MOCCHI. L'influensa del tabagismo sulla gravidansa. Ann d'Obst. e. Gin. 28, 287, N. 2 (cit. NICE).

1923. Z. MORGENSTERN. Zur Frage des morphologischen Verhaltens des Hodens bei akuten Infektionskrankheiten. VIRCHOW's Archiv, 245, 229.

1904. F. NIOSI. L'ovario, etc. negli avuel. da arsenico, mercuro, l'alcool. Ann. d'obst. e. Gin. 26, 677. N. 1 (cit. NICE).

1911. Sir THOMAS OLIVER. A lecture on lead poisoning and the race. Del. to Eug. Ed. Soc. Brit. med. Journ. I, 1096.

1891. H. OPPENHEIM. Allgem. u. Spez. über die toxischen Erkrankungen des Nervensystems. Berl. klin. Wochenschr. Nr. 49.

1913. K. OPPERMANN. Die Entwicklung von Forelleneiern nachBefruchtung mit radiumbestrahlten Samenfäden. S. 141 en 307. Arch. f. mikr. Anat. 2. Abt. 83. Bd.

1930. O. PANKOW. Keimschädigungen durch Röntgenstrahlen. M. m. W. 77, 303. N. 8.

1860. C. PAUL. Etude sur l'intoxication lente par les préparations de plomb, de son influence sur le produit de la conception. Arch. gén. de méd. Vol. I, p. 513 (5e sér. t. 15).

1893. F. M. POPE. Two cases of poisoning by the selfadministration of diachylon lead-plaster — for the purpose of procuring abortion. Brit. med. Journ. 1893, p. 9, Juli 1.

1889. PRÉVOST et BINET. Recherches expér. sur l'intoxication saturnine. Revue suisse Oct., Nov. p. 606, 669 (ref. in VIRCHOW HIRSCH's Jahresbericht über 1889.

1881. RENNERT. Ueb. eine heredit. Form chronischer Bleivergiftigung. Arch. f. Gynaek. (cit. LENZ).

1908. RICHON et PERRIN. Retards de développement par intoxication tabagique expér., etc. Comptes rendus hebd. en mém. de la soc. biol. T. 1 (64), p. 563.

1872. ROQUE. Des dégénérescences hérédit. produites par l'intoxication saturnine lente. C. r. soc. d. biol. 1872, t. IV, p. 243 (cit. DÉJÉRINE).

1927. E. ROST. Borsäure. In Hefter III, 1, S. 456.

1930. Sack und Amersbach. Das Verhalten der menschlichen Spermien gegen Farbstoffe u.s.w. M. med. W. Nr. 10, S. 400.

1929. Starkenstein-Rost-Pohl. Toxicologie.

1924. W. H. Stefko. Über die Veränderungen der Geschlechtsdrüsen des Menschen beim Hungern. Die Sterilisation der Bevölkerung unter dem Einfluss von Hunger. Virchow's Arch. Bd. 229, Bd. 252, S. 385.

1892. L. Stieglitz. Eine experimentelle Untersuchung über Bleivergiftung. Arch. f. Psych. Bd. 24, S. 1.

1926. H. Stieve. Unfruchtbarkeit als Folge unnatürlicher Lebensweise. Grenzfr. Nerv. u. Seelenleb. München. Bergmann.

1928. H. Stieve. Der Einfluss des Coffeins auf die Fortpflanzung des Russenkaninchens. Z. mikr. anat. Forsch. 15, 599.

1930. H. Stieve. Umweltbedingte, nicht durch Röntgenstrahlen veranlasste Keimdrüsenschädigungen. Döderlein-Festschrift. Strahlentherapie 37, 491.

1929. H. Stieve. Kaffeïn und Nachkommenschaft. Med. Welt 1929. Nr. 32, S. 1133, Nr. 33, S. 1173. Cent. allg. Path. u. Path.-anat. 46, Nr. 10.

1907. Ch. R. Stockard. The artif. production of a single median cyclopean eye in the fish embryo, etc. Arch. f. Entw. mech. 23.

1909. Ch. R. Stockard. The development of artificially produced cyclopean fish "the magnesium embryo". Journ. Exp. Zoöl. 6, 285.

1839. L. Tanquerel des Planches. Traité des maladies de plomb. Paris.

1905. Tardieu. Report on Industrial Poisons French Department of Labor (cit. Oliver).

1903. E. Teichmann. Ueb. Furchung befruchteter Seeigeleier u.s.w. Jenaische Zeitschr. f. Nat. wiss. 73, 105.

1919. H. Treub. Leerboek der Verloskunde. Pathologie der zwangerschap, p. 342, 454.

1910. O. Warburg. Ueber die Oxydationen in lebenden Zellen nach Versuchen am Seeïgelei. Zeitschr. f. physiol. Chemie. 66. Bd., S. 305.

1915. C. V. Weller. The blastophthoric effect of chronic lead poisoning. The Journal of med. res. Vol. 33, p. 271. (Also: Proc. Soc. exper. biol. med. 12, 157, 1914).

1928. J. Yamane und K. Kato. Ueber die Befruchtungsfähigkeit der in der mit Phosphat gepufferten Dextroselösung konservierten Spermatozoen beim Kaninchen. Biol. Cent. 48, 459.

1923. Yoshio Yamasaki. Experimentelle Untersuchungen über den Einfluss des Vitamin- oder Zellsalzmangels auf die Entwicklung von Spermatozoën und Eiern. Virchow's Archiv. 245, 513.

1927. W. C. Young. The influence of high temperature on the histology and reproductive capacity of the guinea-pig testis. Anat. Rec. 37, 2, p. 131. Archiv für Gyn. 131, 2, S. 364.

1908. E. von Zebrowski. Zur Frage vom Einfluss des Tabakrauches auf Tiere. Cent. f. Allgem. Path. u. Path.-Anat. 19, S. 609.

1908. Th. Ziehen. Psychiatrie.

1899. W. Zinn. Ueber acute Bleivergiftung. Berl. klin. Woch. Nr. 50, S. 1093.

INDEX OF AUTHORS

ADDENDA

cf. Alcohol, p. 97. STIEVE (1926) gives mice alcohol in the food. Young animals are very sensible, adult ones are less sensible. Adult mice show no changes, — there is a normal offspring —, when they receive 10—20 % alcohol, agreeing on 5—10 g alcohol per 1 Kilo bodyweight. The animals, especially white mice, died after 6 or 7 weeks, when STIEVE gave 30—40 % alcohol. After a few days these animals are impotent and the testicles show important changes. The animals recover soon, when they receive no more alcohol; four weeks later they are fit again for procreation and the offspring is normal.

cf. Lead, p. 117. STIEVE and SCHMIDT (STIEVE 1926) found no changes of the testicles and ovaries of rabbits, that had received large quantities of lead during many weeks.

cf. Morphium, p. 129. Lengthy use of morphium leads to sexual impotency with man, to stagnancy of ovulation with woman after MÜLLER (1924). He mentions two cases, where the children of morphinists were idiots (cit. STIEVE 1926).

1926 H. STIEVE. Unfruchtbarkeit als Folge unnatürlicher Lebensweise. Grenzfragen d. Nerv. u. Seelenlebens. J. F. Bergmann. München.

1930 H. STIEVE. Die temporäre Röntgen amenorrhoe. Strahlentherapie 37, 491.